A UNIQUE RATING SYSTEM THAT INTERPRETS THE DATA INSTANTLY!

Major food group

Handy everyday serving sizes

Fruits, Vegetables, Nuts & Seeds
Vegetables, Frozen, Cooked

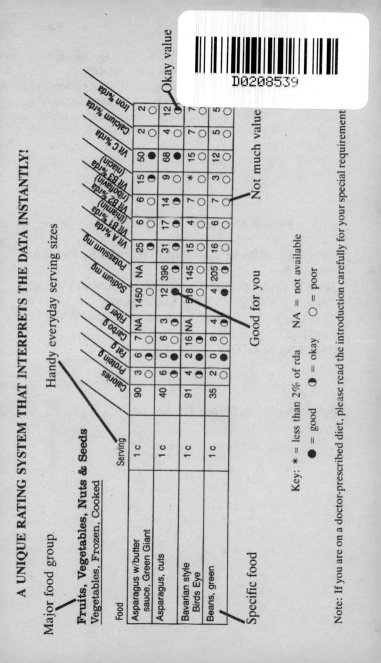

Food	Serving	Calories	Protein g	Fat g	Carbo g	Fiber g	Sodium mg	Potassium mg	Vit A %rda	Vit B1 %rda (thiamin)	Vit B2 %rda (riboflavin)	Vit B3 %rda (niacin)	Vit C %rda	Calcium %rda	Iron %rda
Asparagus w/butter sauce, Green Giant	1 c	90	3	6	7	NA	1450	NA	25	6	6	15	50	2	2
Asparagus, cuts	1 c	40	6	0	3	3	12	396	31	17	14	9	68	4	12
Bavarian style Birds Eye	1 c	91	4	16	2	NA	518	145	15	4	7	*	15	7	7
Beans, green	1 c	35	2	0	8	4	4	205	16	6	7	3	12	5	5

Okay value

Not much value

Good for you

Specific food

Key: * = less than 2% of rda   NA = not available

● = good   ● = okay   ○ = poor

Note: If you are on a doctor-prescribed diet, please read the introduction carefully for your special requirement

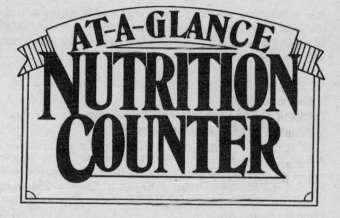

AT-A-GLANCE NUTRITION COUNTER

PATRICIA HAUSMAN

BALLANTINE BOOKS • NEW YORK

A Ballantine Book
Published by The Ballantine Publishing Group
Copyright © 1984 by Patricia Hausman

http://www.randomhouse.com

Library of Congress Catalog Card Number: 84-91046

ISBN 0-345-31183-3

Manufactured in the United States of America

First Ballantine Books Edition: September 1984

OPM 38 37 36 35 34 33 32 31 30 29

to Glenn

Acknowledgments

It took an all-star cast to create the *At-A-Glance Nutrition Counter*. I'd like to introduce the team.

- Marilyn Abraham and Virginia Faber, my editors at Ballantine Books

- Ernest Chesnutis and Rae Dasher, data entry experts who entered the nutrition information into the computer with unprecedented speed, accuracy, and good cheer

- Susan Cohen and Richard Curtis, agents extraordinaire, who attended to countless details

- Glenn Marcus, computer whiz and unsung hero, who designed and developed the amazing nutrient database and computer programs on which this book is based

I also consulted many sources for the nutrition information in this book, among them:

- The Nutrient Data Research Group of the U.S. Department of Agriculture, which supplied data on basic foods

- Dr. James Anderson and staff at the High Carbohydrate and Fiber Research Foundation, who provided some of the fiber information used in our calculations

- Bonnie Liebman, staff nutritionist at the Center for Science in the Public Interest, who compiled some of the sodium values, and

- more than a hundred food companies who responded to my requests for nutrition information on their products

Many thanks to all!

Patricia Hausman
Silver Spring, Maryland
December, 1983

Contents •

Part I

Fruits, Vegetables, Nuts, and Seeds 73

Grain Products 98

Odds and Ends

Combination Foods

Fast Foods

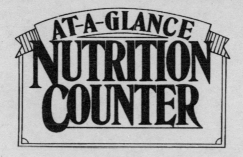

Part I •

Chapter 1 ●
Facts at
Your Fingertips

Nothing makes getting out of bed each morning easier than those tempting aromas that come only from the kitchen. But better yet is knowing that the food that awaits you is not only delicious, but healthful too.

That's where the *At-A-Glance Nutrition Counter* comes in. It's designed to help you separate the nourishing foods from the not-so-nourishing ones—without spending half the day doing so.

It's my answer to the question that the mailman so often brings me in letters from my readers. "Why can't you nutritionists make nutrition simpler?", they ask.

The letters are always from people who care deeply about their health. But they have found that staying informed about good nutrition has become too time-consuming.

It is not hard to understand why. Today, food shoppers have about 10,000 products to choose from and about three dozen nutrients to consider. Trying to keep tabs on so many foods is no simple task—not even for those of us trained in nutrition.

Getting Started

One day, while reading one of my favorite medical journals, I found my mind wandering back to the idea of simplifying nutrition. I put the technical reading aside and jotted down a few "musts."

Here is what I wrote:

- put all of the important information on basic and brand name foods in one book
- include ethnic foods and restaurant items, such as those served in fast food outlets
- translate the endless string of nutrient values into simple terms, such as good, okay, or poor
- offer a handy guide to the best and worst Foods for sodium, fat, and other nutrients of major concern
- list values for fiber, so hard to come by, even today
- use meaningful serving sizes, like one cup, instead of 100 grams or 3.5 ounces
- use only the latest, most up-to-date information available
- express vitamin and mineral levels as a percentage of the U.S. Recommended Daily Allowances, not in milligrams
- maintain enough detail to help those on special diets
- expose and correct deceptive tactics occasionally used to make foods look more healthful than they are

The *At-A-Glance Nutrition Counter* was born.

Taming the Numbers

Those were my ten commandments. They never changed during the many months that I spent preparing this book.

I never doubted which goal meant most to me. More than anything, I wanted to offer an alternative to all of the numbers that grace food labels and books about nutrition.

Yet, I knew that some people need these numbers. If you are one of the many people on a low-sodium diet, for instance, you may need to know precisely how much sodium a food contains—not simply that it is low, medium, or high in this substance.

So I decided to give you the best of both worlds. In this book, you can choose between two lines of information for each food. The first line offers the classic approach—numbers. *The second line is the at-a-glance line.* It rates the food's level of each nutrient as good, okay, or poor. Instead of words, I use simple symbols.

- (●) means good
- (◑) means okay
- (○) means poor

Unless your needs differ from those of most people, good means that, for the nutrient in question, the food is good for you. For the most part, this means that the food is high in a nutrient. *But fat and sodium are exceptions to this rule. The good symbol in the fat and sodium columns means that the food is low in these two trouble-makers*; again this means good for most people's health.

For carbohydrates, good means that the food is a good source of complex carbohydrates, also known as starches. (Contrary to former beliefs, these starches are good for us!)

Conversely, the poor symbol usually means that the food contains no, or small amounts of, a vitamin, mineral, or protein. *Again, fat and sodium are exceptions. The poor symbol alerts you to foods that are high in fat or sodium.* The poor symbol in the carbohydrate column means that the food is high in added sugar, or that it contains little of the nourishing starches.

The okay symbol means that the food has an average content of protein, vitamins, calcium, or iron; when used in the carbohydrate column, it indicates a moderate level of starches or sugar. For fat and sodium, this symbol tells you that the food contains reasonable, though not low, amounts of these substances.

Are the At-A-Glance Ratings for You?

Much as I like the simplicity of the rating system, I must tell you emphatically that it is not appropriate for everyone.

The rating system is designed to conform to the federal government's Dietary Guidelines for Americans. The Guidelines advise us to eat adequate amounts of starches and fiber, and to avoid high levels of sodium, fat, and cholesterol.

In addition, the Guidelines stress variety, to allow a healthy intake of vitamins, minerals, and protein.

Some people, however, are on special diets that contradict the Guidelines. Protein, iron, and potassium, for instance, are usually considered healthful nutrients. The rating system rewards foods containing high levels of them.

If you are a kidney patient, or have an iron storage disease, however, you may have been advised to avoid foods rich in these substances. If you have a gastrointestinal disorder, you may be limiting, not increasing, your fiber intake.

The *At-A-Glance Nutrition Counter* can make following special diets such as these much easier. *But you must use only the numerical values, not the at-a-glance line, for any nutrient for which your needs differ from those of the general public.*

My rating system aside, I would like to tell you how the *At-A-Glance Nutrition Counter* fulfills my other goals for simplifying nutrition.

The Road to Simplicity

As a professional nutritionist, I knew where to start collecting facts that I wanted to put at your fingertips. Nutritionists turn first to the U.S. Department of Agriculture (USDA) for nutrition information. It publishes food tables showing the nutritional value of hundreds of basic foods: fruits, vegetables, dairy products, and meats.

I entered much of the USDA's information into my computer. That accomplished, I could easily find the protein, vitamin, and mineral content of common foods.

But when I finished putting all of the available facts into the computer, I still had that sinking feeling that my work was far from finished. For one thing, half the foods in my kitchen were not listed in the USDA tables. What's more, the information from the USDA was clearly designed with the nutritionist, not the consumer, in mind.

Breaking the Brand Name Barrier

I have great respect for the nutrition information that the USDA provides. Criticizing it is not easy. But I do have a few complaints.

For starters, I wish I knew where the USDA got the idea that nice girls don't use brand names. Instead of listing foods by the familiar names, the USDA gives long descriptions such as:

- honeycombed hard candy with peanut butter
- white bread, enriched, soft-crumb type made by continuous mix or conventional method
- bran with added sugar, salt, defatted wheat germ, vitamins

It has always been a challenge for me to figure out which product the USDA is talking about. In some cases, I never have.

My food tables, I decided, would call a spade a spade. But rather than second-guess the USDA, I simply asked scores of food companies to provide me with nutrition information for their products. That way I did not risk attaching the wrong brand name to the USDA descriptions.

So you will not find any longwinded euphemisms in this book. I call a Milky Way a Milky Way.

Keeping Up-to-Date

The most popular USDA food tables, Handbooks 8 and 456, are based on studies done in 1963. About five years ago, the USDA began the overwhelming job of updating its numbers.

How things have changed since 1963! The fat content of chicken, for instance, has jumped, while the iron content of beef and pork has been lower in recent studies than in the 1963 analysis.

Whenever possible, I used the USDA's revised information. But since many packaged foods have yet to be re-analyzed, I relied on numbers from food companies whenever possible. Often, these figures are more recent, and giving you the most up-to-date information is one of my goals. I used the latest information available to me when I began this project in 1982.

For packaged foods, I favor the food manufacturer's nutrition information for another reason. Sodium content often varies from one brand to another of the same product—by as much as 300 per cent.

For this reason, it's better to get the facts from the manufacturer. They know best how much sodium they put in there.

What's more, you can do comparison shopping. I have made it easy to see which brand of popular items boasts the lowest sodium count.

Combinations without Calculations

Variety is the spice of life, we say, and the notion applies very well to food. Few of us would want to part with the great variety of foods in today's supermarket.

Much of these items are combinations of basic foods—be it pasta with tomato sauce and cheese, broccoli with onions and cream sauce . . . the list of combinations goes on and on.

But who wants to sit around adding the sodium in the tomato sauce and the pasta to the sodium in the cheese, and so on for each nutrient that's important. That is why I have a section called Combination Foods. It gives you the final tallies for the dozens of combination foods that are often on the menu.

In addition, I have included an extensive section entitled Fast Foods. It provides nutrient information for dozens of sandwiches and platters served at the ever-popular fast food outlets. This way, you don't have to add the calories in a hamburger bun, ground beef patty, and cheese to know the caloric count of your cheeseburger.

Accent on Ethnic Foods

I have not forgotten ethnic foods either. From whitefish to wonton soup, chili to chow mein, they are here. See the Ethnic Dishes section, under Combination Foods, for the profile on such favorites as:

- burritos and refried beans
- egg rolls and chow mein
- ethnic soups
- pierogies, the Polish dumplings
- matzoh, gefilte fish, and borscht
- tacos, tamales and fritters

Making Sense of Serving Sizes

Some food companies do a fantastic job of analyzing the protein, vitamin, and mineral content of their products. Then they blow it by describing the portion size in terms that even nutritionists can hardly picture.

I have a master's degree in nutrition, but I honestly don't find it very useful to read that 3½ ounces of peas has five grams of protein. It has never occurred to me to weigh my peas before eating them.

We usually judge portion size with our eyes, not with scales. So, whenever possible, I have translated serving sizes from ounces to a measure you can visualize. Usually it is cups.

Doing this took some letter-writing to food companies, but it was definitely worth it. I can now make sense of nutrition information that was once all but useless to me.

For meats and frozen entrees, however, I had to abandon

my principles and use ounces. It is simpler to say four ounces of roast beef than to describe the length, width, and thickness of a dozen pieces of meat all weighing this amount.

Likewise, frozen entrees often come in packages containing a single serving. I thought it simpler to say one 7-ounce package of a product than to translate the weight into cups.

Keeping Serving Sizes Consistent

Another important feature of the *At-A-Glance Nutrition Counter* is *standard serving sizes within each category of food whenever possible.*

The original nutrition information for juices from frozen concentrates, for instance, measured some as ¾ cup, other types as one cup, and still others as ½ cup. I converted all of them to one cup. Now you can easily choose the lowest calorie juice, or the one richest in vitamin C.

I want you to know that making these changes did require a trade-off. Food companies round off their nutrition information to comply with federal regulations. A value such as 64, for instance, would be rounded down to 60; 66 would be rounded up to 70. This means that the numbers can vary from the true value by up to 5% of the RDA.

When I increased the serving sizes of some foods, the amount of rounding may have increased somewhat also. But after much thought, I concluded that the benefits of standard serving sizes outweighed this disadvantage. The computer was programmed to spot cases where changing the serving size chosen by the manufacturer might result in numbers too far from the true value. In these cases, the manufacturer's serving size was left unchanged.

I also found some categories of foods where it didn't make sense to use the same serving size for all items. Alcoholic beverages are a case in point. We drink beer by the 12-ounce bottle or can, not by the cup. The usual serving size for wine, on the other hand, is just under a half cup. Converting wine and beer to one cup, when we don't serve them that way, would not have made sense.

Likewise, breakfast cereals such as granolas, are very dense, while puffed cereals are the opposite. Eating a cup of puffed cereal is easy, but a full cup of granola is probably more than you'd eat at a meal. For this reason, I've used three standards for cereals:

- very dense cereals are measured as ⅓ cup
- flake cereals are measured as ⅔ cup
- puffed cereals and other very light varieties have been standardized to one cup each

Items such as cocoa mixes and oatmeal often come in packets. One manufacturer's packet yields a cup of cocoa, while another's makes only ¾ cup. Again, I stayed with the manufacturer's serving size in these cases. It was the only sensible thing to do.

Games Food Companies Play

Most food companies provide their nutrition information in good faith. They deserve credit for their responsiveness to you, the consumer, who wants food that nourishes the body as well as the palate.

Sad to say, a few food companies resort to deceptive tactics in their nutrition information. More than one food company, for example, lists sodium in grams. Just 1.4 grams of sodium per serving? A great food for sodium-watchers, no?

No way. Surely that food company knows that sodium should be measured in milligrams, not grams. That value should read a whopping 1400 milligrams, not 1.4 grams. In this book, it does.

Just the same, manufacturers of stuffing mixes know that we add margarine or butter to them before eating. Why, then, does a major company offer us nutrition information only for the dry crumbs? Perhaps because the calorie content jumps by 50% when butter is added?

Not to mention the company that sends nutrition information for its products based on a realistic one-ounce portion. Sodium, however, is listed on separate pages, for *half-ounce* portions. A clever way to make the foods look only half as bad? Don't fall for it.

In this book, I have uncloaked all misrepresentations such as these. That meant changing one gram to 1000 milligrams, doubling sodium values where serving sizes had been halved, and adjusting calorie, fat, and sodium values to include margarine or butter added during preparation. I am also looking forward to the day when the companies involved get with it and give us the facts straight.

Finding the Fiber Content

Fiber is one of top-rated nutrients these days. But strangely enough, hard facts about the fiber content of foods are tough to come by. The USDA's authorities on food composition aren't even measuring it for their new food tables.

It is no surprise, then, that most food companies are also mum on the subject. They often blame the scientists, who have been debating how to measure fiber for almost a decade now.

But the good news is that a few researchers have been hard at work analyzing the fiber content of food. Their results are often buried deep in medical journals, but I've dug them out for you. In this book you'll find facts on fiber for most basic foods, and for breakfast cereals.

By the way, don't confuse crude fiber with dietary fiber. Crude fiber includes only some of the various forms of fiber in food.

Until recently, crude fiber was considered a rough guide to the total fiber content of food. But researchers laid this notion to rest a few years ago. They have shown that crude fiber is not proportional to the total fiber in food. Your best bet is to ignore crude fiber values. That is what I do.

Fiber, by the way, is one of the nutrients for which you can find a chart listing the best sources. See Chapter 5.

Simplicity Isn't Everything

After spending months and months working to simplify nutrition, I have never forgotten that sometimes simplicity has a price.

At the turn of the century, for instance, nutrition couldn't have been simpler. Scientists knew that food contains protein, carbohydrate, fat, and a few minerals. That was nutrition, in a nutshell.

The word vitamin wasn't even in the dictionary then. Scientists had no idea that food contained more than a dozen vitamins that safeguarded health.

Nor had they any idea that the fiber in food helped them to stay healthy. They weren't watching their sodium intake, or their fat intake.

But ignorance was hardly bliss. Nutrient deficiencies such as scurvy and pellagra haunted the globe, killing thousands of people. There was little hope for diabetics. Heart disease and cancer were accepted as inevitable—the price to pay for growing old.

Thanks to nutrition research, the picture has changed dramatically. The statisticians who tally up disease figures each year can count the number of scurvy victims in the United States on one hand.

And scurvy isn't the only disease on the decline. Heart disease rates are down too, in recent years, thanks partly to better diets that contain less saturated fat and cholesterol. New knowledge about diet and diabetes, not to mention invaluable drugs, have added years to the life expectancy of diabetics.

Most heartening of all, scientists no longer accept cancer as man's fate. Again, nutrition is in the spotlight. Research links diets low in fat and rich in fiber, vitamin C, and carotene (a form of vitamin A) to less chance of developing cancer.

Today, nutrition is more complicated, but also more exciting than it has ever been. Much as I want to simplify nutrition, I don't long for the old days when simplicity meant too little knowledge about the nutrients in food and their role in good health.

I hope you'll agree that nutrition should not be so simple that important nutrients are overlooked. That's why this book contains thirteen nutrients, plus calories, not to mention more than 1500 different foods.

If you do agree with me, keep this book handy. It can help you reap the tremendous rewards that good nutrition can bring.

Chapter 2●
Finding What
You Want

Now that you know why I wrote this book, let me offer some pointers about making it work for you.

As the Contents show, this book contains nine broad categories:

- Beverages
- Dairy and Eggs
- Fruits, Vegetables, Nuts & Seeds
- Grain Products
- Meat, Poultry, & Fish
- Sweets & Snacks
- Miscellaneous
- Combination Foods
- Fast Foods

To make locating foods easier, I have divided the main groups into subgroups. Sweets & Snacks, for instance, has separate sections on cakes, cookies, pies, puddings, snacks, sugars, and syrups.

You will probably find most foods that interest you simply by checking the logical subgroup.

One note about ethnic foods. In general, staples such as beans, are usually not classified under Ethnic Dishes. Only combinations of ingredients fall under this category.

The reason is simple: Chinese cabbage isn't always used in an ethnic dish, nor are beans. Look for individual items such as these under basic food categories. When in doubt, check the index.

The Importance of the Headings

To use the *At-A-Glance Nutrition Counter*, keep one rule in mind. Always check the category heading as you run through the pages.

Here's why. I didn't want to repeat the word pie for every flavor of pie in the book. Instead, I have a section headed Pies. Each entry below it lists only the flavor—the word pie is not repeated.

Therefore, if you randomly open to any page of this book, and find a food entry that reads "peach," you need to check the category heading. That will let you know whether the listing refers to a fresh peach, frozen peaches, canned peaches, or peach pie.

Within Each Category

Within each group, foods are arranged as follows:

- If the food name begins with a symbol, it will be among the first items under the heading.
  Example: $100,000 bar is the first item listed under Candy, because it begins with a symbol rather than a number or letter.
- Food names that begin with a number come after those starting with a symbol and before names that begin with letters.
  Example: 3 Musketeers follows the $100,000 bar under Candy, yet precedes Almond Joy, which begins with a letter.
- Once the food names beginning with letters appear, each is listed alphabetically.

Flavor names, such as apple or cherry, usually are not considered the first word of the food name. For instance, apple Danish is not listed that way, but as "Danish, apple." That way, all flavors of Danishes appear together, not scattered throughout the Pastry section.

Picking Package Sizes

Food companies often offer their products in more than one size. When this is the case, I show the package weight or volume of the package I'm referring to. This appears within the food description.

Some serving sizes appear in a format slightly different than shown by the manufacturer. This was done so that we could convert serving sizes to standard amounts. For example, an amount such as 1¼ cups has been changed to 1.25 cups.

For simplicity, all values shown in the charts have been rounded to one decimal place. Therefore, the package label might read 9.55 ounces. In this book, that will be listed as 9.6 ounces. I tell you this so that you will know that we are talking about the same product even though the weight or cups might be recorded a little bit differently.

About Mixes and Reconstituted Products

As I mentioned in Chapter 1, I think it is misleading when food companies provide nutrition information for their products as packaged, but not as prepared.

Almost without exception, the information in this book applies to the product *when prepared as directed*. In other words, for cake mixes, sauce mixes, cocoa mixes, and the like, the values represent the prepared item after other ingredients are added. Here are some important examples:

- Soup listings for condensed or powdered products include water added during preparation.

- Puddings refer to products after addition of the type of milk recommended on the label.
- Milk flavorings, such as Quik and Instant Slender, are not listed as powders, but as Flavored Milks. The values represent the nutritional value of the food after adding the type of milk recommended on the label.

Two notable exceptions to this rule. Listings for cold cereals do not include added milk. Powdered seasonings (for meat, fish, and tacos) listed under Condiments refer to the product as packaged.

When Asterisks and "NA" Appear

You have probably noticed asterisks on the nutriton information panel of food labels. In this book, as on the food label, an asterisk means that the food contains less than 2% of the U.S. Recommended Daily Allowance for the nutrient in question.

The abbreviation NA stands for not available. Often, manufacturers of brand name foods do not analyze their products for sodium, potassium, or fiber. The Food and Drug Administration has deemed these three as "optional nutrients." Manufacturers that offer nutrition information do not have to give values for these three nutrients.

With no law that these values be disclosed, some companies choose to stay quiet, particularly on the subject of sodium. More often than not, when the manufacturer will not disclose the sodium content, the level is quite high. If you are on a low-sodium diet, don't take chances; avoid those products for which no sodium information is available.

Occasionally, the sodium content of a product will vary slightly among different flavors. When this happens, the food table shows the sodium content of the flavor containing the most sodium. For instance, if the strawberry flavor of a product contains 60 milligrams of sodium, while the chocolate flavor has 55, the food table will simply show 60, the higher value.

However, if the variation is substantial, each flavor appears separately, with its exact sodium content.

Sometimes, food companies list nutrient levels as "less than 10" or another number. In this case, I simply used the next lower number. That is, "less than 10" would appear in the table as 9.

Table of Equivalents

There's one more thing you might want to know about the tables: how to convert from one measure (such as cups) to another (such as tablespoons). The table below shows you how.

$$1 \text{ cup} = 16 \text{ tablespoons}$$
$$1 \text{ tablespoon} = 3 \text{ teaspoons}$$
$$1 \text{ fluid ounce (fl. oz.)} = 2 \text{ tablespoons of liquids}$$
$$1 \text{ fluid ounce (fl. oz.)} = 6 \text{ teaspoons of liquids}$$
$$1 \text{ cup of liquids} = 8 \text{ fluid ounces}$$

Chapter 3 •
Choosing The Right
Stuff for You

The *At-A-Glance Nutrition Counter* lists thirteen nutrients, in addition to calories. It's fun to skim through the book and see the all-star foods—the ones that rate "good" on most or all counts.

I did not intend for you to monitor your intake of each of these nutrients, though. Rather, I hope you will use this book to track the nutrients most important to *your* health.

Chances are that you are already on the look-out for one or more nutrients. The following sections will help you determine which, if any, others are especially important for you.

For Weight Control

The *At-A-Glance Nutrition Counter* makes calorie counters obsolete. It's not that calories don't matter—they do. But newer knowledge hints that other nutrients can help with weight control, too.

Most important, perhaps, is fiber. Research has found that fiber can interfere with the body's absorption of the calories in food. It's only a slight effect; people on high-fiber diets seem to absorb about 1–3% fewer calories than those on low-fiber diets. But though the number seems small, it might make the difference between gaining a few pounds every year, or staying at the same weight.

Though fiber information is unavailable for many name brand foods, I have been able to provide it for most basic foods. I know it will be useful.

When you tire of calorie-counting, you might simply watch your fat intake instead. Fat, not carbohydrate, is what makes your calorie intake soar. Each gram of fat in food has nine calories; each gram of carbohydrate only four. The numbers make clear that cutting back on fat is the best way to cut calories.

How about carbohydrates and weight control? Actually, low-carbohydrate diets are rarely a good way to lose weight. These diets cause a rapid weight loss at first that is mostly water, not body fat. The water weight returns once you resume normal carbohydrate intake.

What's more, these diets can be dangerously high in fat and cholesterol. I never have recommended them, and probably never will. However, if you feel you have a good reason to watch your carbohydrate intake, this book will give you the facts you need to do it.

For Your Heart's Content

If you have high blood pressure, you may be on a low-sodium diet. The sodium column of this book will make your job a lot easier.

You may also be taking medication for your blood pressure that lowers your body's supply of potassium. Your doctor may have advised you to eat foods rich in potassium. If so, take a good look at the potassium column.

Watching your fat intake may also help control your blood pressure. Some scientists believe that high fat diets may play a role in some forms of high blood pressure. If they are right, the culprit is probably saturated fat, not the poly-unsaturated fat that abounds in vegetable oils.

Meat and dairy fats, as well as coconut oil, palm oil, and some vegetable shortenings, are high in saturated fats. Since most high-fat foods are high in saturated fat, keeping your eyes on the fat column of this book will help you ferret saturated fat from your diet.

But even if fat has no effect on blood pressure, it has plenty of effect on your heart. Saturated fats raise the blood cholesterol level, and as it rises, so do your chances of suffering a heart attack.

So heart-watchers, take heed. To keep the heart healthy, feast on lowfat foods. To find them, just look down the fat column for the good symbol. It lets you pick out the lowfat foods at a glance.

Saturated fat is by far the most important influence on blood cholesterol. But new research shows that a healthy intake of some forms of fiber can help control blood cholesterol. For the most part, it's the fiber in fruits, vegetables, beans, and oats that seems to lower cholesterol.

You probably need to eat about six servings a day of these foods to have an effect. It's well worth doing so, because these foods have still other virtues. Research links nutrients in fruits, vegetables, and whole grain foods to reduced risk of cancer. Read the next section for the story.

For Cancer Prevention

The most exciting news in nutrition is about cancer prevention. Impressive studies the world over have convinced cancer scientists (and me!) that certain nutrients may help protect us from common forms of cancer. For the complete picture, see *Foods That Fight Cancer*, my book on this subject.

Three nutrients are in the spotlight as *protective elements*. They are:

- carotene, the main form of vitamin A in fruits and vegetables
- vitamin C, which occurs mostly in fruits and vegetables
- fiber in some forms (mainly those that occur in whole grain foods)

In addition, research strongly links diets low in fat to low rates of breast, colon, and prostate cancers.

At the request of the federal government's National Cancer Institute, the National Academy of Sciences reviewed all of the research on nutrition and cancer prevention. In 1982, the Academy's blue-ribbon Committee on Diet, Nutrition, and Cancer issued its recommendations. The group urged us to eat more fruits and vegetables rich in vitamins A and C, and to eat whole grain foods daily. They also advised us to eat less fat.

The *At-A-Glance Nutrition Counter* makes it easy to follow this advice. Take a glance at the fruit and vegetable sections to find those items high in vitamin A or C (often the same foods). Then turn to the bread and cereal sections and learn which items are high in whole grain fiber. Finally, keep your eye on the fat column, emphasizing the foods that rate "good." These lowfat items should be the backbone of your diet.

Some high-fat foods are among Americans' favorites. You don't have to give them up, just eat fewer of them. Eating no more than two servings of high-fat foods a day isn't difficult. Your health is worth it.

Especially for Women

If you're a woman, the last two columns of the *At-A-Glance Nutrition Counter* are especially for you. They contain information about two important minerals: calcium and iron.

Men need calcium and iron, too, but women are most likely to suffer the ill effects of low-calcium diets. The results of too little can be mild to devastating.

Too little calcium catches up with women after menopause, in the form of osteoporosis. This condition causes loss of calcium from the bones. In turn, the bones become brittle and easily broken. This is no rare disease in the U.S. Thousands of women suffer from it.

Start on the road to prevention today. A quick glance down the calcium column will show you the leaders for this mineral. Eat more of them.

As for iron, the body does its best to hang on to the iron absorbed from food. But iron does much of its work in the blood, and when blood is lost, so is this nutrient.

Menstruation, of course, results in loss of blood. Iron goes with it. That's why, like calcium, iron is especially important for women.

Though women need more iron than men, they usually get less of it in their diets. The reason is simple: women eat fewer calories than men do, and a lower calorie intake usually means a lower iron intake.

Vitamin C can help your body make the most of the iron you eat. Studies show that vitamin C helps the body to absorb iron. So the vitamin C column of this book deserves as much attention as does the iron column.

How can you know whether you are low on iron? A simple blood test will tell your doctor whether you are. If so, keep your eyes on the vitamin C and iron columns, and keep your kitchen stocked with foods rich in them.

Chapter 4 ●
Your Questions
Answered

As I developed the *At-A-Glance Nutrition Counter*, I was careful to ask consumers for feedback. Their comments on the nutrient tables have enabled me to present nutrition information in the best way possible.

As I listened to consumers' opinions, I noticed that many asked the same questions about the nutrition information in the book. Chances are that you, too, may have one or more of the same questions. That's why I have devoted this section to answering the most common questions asked of me.

Here they are.

How did you determine cut-off points between good and okay, okay and poor?

Designing the rating system was a major step for us. We first considered human needs for the nutrient. Then we had the computer analyze the availability of each nutrient in the food supply. This provided the basis for dividing foods into three categories—good, okay, and poor—for most of the nutrients.

Sodium required a different approach, because most of it is added by food companies, not put there by nature. I based the sodium ratings on amounts that would be likely to keep your sodium intake within the level now recommended for the general public. The numbers are as follows. Please note that these ratings are not stringent enough for those on strict low-sodium diets.

(●): less than 100 milligrams
(◑): 100–325 milligrams
(○): more than 325 milligrams

In designing the ratings for fat, I also drew the dividing lines somewhat differently. In addition to the computer's print-out showing how fat is distributed in the food supply, I also estimated the amounts that would enable you to meet official recommendations calling for a 25% drop in fat intake. The rating system is designed accordingly.

If you base your diet mostly on foods that have a good or okay rating for fat, you are probably enjoying a diet that conforms to the recommendations of our most distinguished scientists.

Why aren't calories rated?

If one food has 10% more of a vitamin or mineral than another, the difference is insignificant for most people. But the calorie count is an exception.

Most of us gain weight slowly, by consuming 1 or 2% more calories than we burn up. These small differences can add up as the months and years go by.

Since twenty or so calories can make a difference over a long period of time, I did not want a food with 200 calories per serving to have the same rating as a food having 220 calories per serving. That is why only the calorie count is listed for each food.

Why should I have to go through your book to find nutrition information. Why doesn't it appear on all food labels?

Nutrition labeling is strictly voluntary, and it probably always will be. Congress has never been close to requiring this information on food labels.

The Food and Drug Administration does have regulations on nutrition labeling for those companies that do choose to provide it. Unfortunately, the rules leave something to be desired. There is nothing, for instance, to stop food companies from playing the games described in Chapter 1 in order to deceive consumers about a food's healthfulness.

I have compiled this book to fill the void left by the government's unwillingness to require useful nutrition information on food labels. I have a dream that someday all labels will bear this information. But it is not a dream that I am expecting to come true.

Food labels often give some of the nutrition information I want, but not all of it. I want to keep my heart healthy, so the most important information for me is sodium, saturated fat, and cholesterol. Why do nutrition labels tell me about vitamins that I don't care about, and skip the really important facts?

Powerful industries and farm groups have vehemently opposed proposals to require this information on food labels.

As noted above, food manufacturers don't have to provide any nutrition information at all. But if they do, certain nutrients must be listed. Unfortunately, or perhaps outrageously, saturated fat, cholesterol, and sodium aren't among the required nutrients. You can be sure that political pressures played a role in the FDA's decision to make these three "optional" nutrients.

Every now and then I do find a label that provides the cholesterol content of the food. Then there is a line saying "Information on fat and cholesterol content is provided for individuals, who, on the advice of a physician, are modifying their total dietary intake of fat and/or cholesterol." I thought the government itself had advised us to reduce our fat and cholesterol intake. Why the doubletalk?

You're absolutely right. This disclaimer, required by the FDA when cholesterol content appears, is silly. Implying that you should only watch your fat and cholesterol intake on your doctor's advice is like saying that you should smoke cigarettes unless your doctor tells you otherwise.

This disclaimer keeps the meat, dairy, and egg lobbies happy, but it contradicts the government's own advice to all healthy Americans. That advice, contained in the U.S. Dietary Guidelines for Americans, recommends that we all avoid diets high in fat and cholesterol.

Nutrition labels claim to give a food's percentage of the Recommended Dietary Allowances for various vitamins and minerals. Aren't there several sets of RDAs, depending on your age and sex? Which set of RDAs are used to compute the numbers shown on food labels?

Nutrition scientists affiliated with the National Academy of Sciences devise the Recommended Dietary Allowances, and they give sixteen sets of them. There are two sets for infants, three for children, and eleven for teenagers and adults of various ages. Lactating women have still another set.

Obviously, food companies don't have room on the label to give the percent of RDA for each age and sex group. Instead, they use a set of RDA prescribed by the FDA. To minimize confusion, the FDA's values are called the U.S. RDA. (For reasons that are beyond me, the FDA has decreed that the term RDA, when used on nutrition labels, stands for Recommended *Daily* Allowances. Everyone else knows that the term RDA, as used by the nutrition profession, is short for Recommended *Dietary* Allowances.)

The FDA sets its U.S. RDA by taking the highest value recommended for any age or sex group. Often, the highest RDA for a nutrient is for teenage boys. That means that the number on food labels (and in this book) basically shows how well the food meets the need of a male teenager.

Children or adult women often need less of a nutrient than a teenage boy. But the U.S. RDA does not reflect this. It makes foods look like they provide less of a child or woman's needs than is actually the case. In other words, the U.S. RDA can be artificially high, depending on how closely your needs resemble those of teenage boys.

Is the U.S. RDA the average need of a teenage boy, the minimum need, or what?

Don't confuse the U.S. RDA—or the National Academy of Sciences' RDA—with the Minimum Daily Requirement from vitamin labels.

The RDA are not a minimum, nor an average. Rather, they are estimates of the most that any healthy individual would need to prevent nutrient deficiencies.

As an example, imagine that you determined the precise amount of protein needed each day by 99 people. From experiments, we know that these needs vary from one person to another.

Armed with the results of your laboratory work, you ask the people to line up in order of their protein needs, with the person needing the least protein first in line. The RDA for the group would not be the level needed by a person in the middle of the line. Rather, it would be the amount needed by the last person in the line.

Obviously, the RDA are deliberately set on the high side. The reasoning goes as follows. If we know that everyone in the group takes in as much protein as the last person in line needs, we can conclude everyone is getting enough. That is the purpose of the RDA—to judge the diet of the group. The RDA are really not intended for evaluating the diets on an individual basis.

How can I tell how close RDA is to   y personal needs?

There is no foolproof way to calculate your own needs, based upon the RDA. Only elaborate laboratory studies can truly measure a person's needs.

You can get an idea of whether your nutrient needs might be more or less than the RDA by comparing your weight to the weight scientists use as the standard for setting the RDA.

For adult women, scientists base their RDA on a women weighing 120 pounds. If you weigh far more, your nutrient needs may be higher. For men, the RDA are based on men weighing 163 pounds. Again, those who weigh far more (or far less) might expect their own needs to vary accordingly.

When I read nutrition labels, it seems that the numbers are always rounded off. I often see 60% or 70% as the percentage of the U.S. RDA, but never see 64% or 68%. Why?

As noted in Chapter 1, the FDA requires food companies to round off their numbers. Levels of 10% or less of the U.S. RDA must be rounded to the nearest even number.

Between 10% and 50% of the RDA, the value must be rounded to the nearest 5-percent level (15, 20, 25, etc). Above 50% of the RDA, the value must be rounded to 60, 70, 80, 90, or 100 percent, whichever is closest. Other values, such as calories and sodium, must likewise be rounded off.

I see no good reason to do this, so I did not round off the numbers like this when I computed the percent of U.S. RDA contained in basic foods. I had no choice but to use these rounded off numbers for the brand name foods, as most manufacturers only offer nutrient levels that have been rounded as prescribed by the FDA.

Didn't the Senate Nutrition Subcommittee issue a report called Dietary Goals for the United States *some time ago? I'd like to have a list of the recommended goals.*

The Senate Nutrition Subcommittee's *Dietary Goals for the United States* was a landmark report that drew enormous attention to contemporary nutrition issues such as fat, cholesterol, sodium, and fiber. The seven goals are as follows:

- If overweight, reduce to normal weight.
- Increase complex carbohydrates and naturally occuring sugars from current level of 28% of total calories to 48% of total calories.
- Reduce refined sugar intake from current level of 18% of total calories to 10% of total calories.
- Reduce fat intake from current level of 42% of calories to 30% of calories.
- Reduce saturated fat intake from current level of 16% of total calories to 10% of calories.
- Reduce cholesterol intake from 600 mg per day to 300 mg per day.
- Limit salt intake to about 5 grams per day, resulting in a sodium intake of about 2000 mg per day.

How to accomplish these goals? To turn theory into practice, the *Dietary Goals* report suggests:

- Eat more fruits, vegetables, and whole grains.
- Eat fewer foods rich in refined sugars.
- Eat fewer high-fat foods and replace some foods rich in saturated fat with polyunsaturated fats.
- Cut down on animal fat and choose meats, poultry, and fish that will reduce saturated-fat intake.
- Except for young children, substitute low-fat and nonfat milk for whole milk, and low-fat dairy products for high-fat dairy products.

- Eat less butterfat, eggs, and other high-cholesterol foods.
- Eat fewer foods rich in sodium and cut back on salt added to food during preparation and at the table.

Chapter 5 ●
The Best and
Worst of . . .

In Chapter 1, I promised to show you the foods that are the best and worst sources of important nutrients. The purpose of this chapter is to fulfill my promise.

The following charts will show you the best sources of the following nutrients:

- fiber
- protein
- potassium

In addition, you'll learn which foods are highest and lowest in fat and sodium.

You should know about a few details. First, by "best" and "worst," I am referring to the best and worst among the more than 1500 foods included in this book. If a food isn't listed in the book, it wasn't included in the analysis of best and worst.

Also, fiber, sodium, and potassium values were not available for every food in the book. If a food is listed in the main charts, but an NA appears for sodium, the food obviously could not be included in the best and worst analyses. Ditto for foods that have NA in the fiber or potassium column.

It made the most sense to divide the best protein foods into three categories: animal foods, vegetable foods, and fast foods.

Fat and sodium presented special problems. So many foods are high in sodium that a list of them all would have gone on for pages. And surprisingly enough, many other foods contain hardly any sodium at all. Again, a list of all foods having less than 10 milligrams of sodium would have taken page after page.

To solve this problem, I have compiled the sodium list by food type. The chart shows you which foods in each class (e.g. canned fruit, cereals, frozen vegetables) are usually low in sodium. *The distinctions of low or high are based on the serving sizes for the food that are shown in the main charts.*

The best and worst charts on fat follow the same approach as the sodium charts. Again, so many foods qualify as very high or very low that a list of every item would cause eyestrain.

Finally, please note that the following abbreviations appear in the charts:

> c = cup(s)
> oz = ounce(s)
> pc = piece(s)
> pr = portion
> sl = slice(s)

High on Fiber

Food	Serving size	Fiber, grams
Kidney beans, canned	1 c	19
Lima beans	1 c	18
Navy beans	1 c	17
Great northern beans	1 c	16
Dates, chopped	1 c	16
Barley, pearled, raw	1 c	13
Peas	1 c	13
Whole wheat flour	1 c	11
Spinach	1 c	11
Raisins	1 c	10
Corn, yellow, plain	1 c	10
Fig, dried, medium	1	9
Raspberries	1 c	9
Corn, yellow	1 c	9
Bran Buds cereal	⅓ c	8
Prunes	5	8
Lentils	1 c	7
Apple, large	1	7
Blackberries	1 c	7
Dates	10	7
Broccoli	1 c	7
Fresh Horizons wheat bread	2 sl	6
100% Bran cereal	⅓ c	6
Bran Chex cereal	⅔ c	6
Oatmeal	1 c	6
Almonds, chopped	⅓ c	6
Broccoli	1 c	6
Parsnips	1 c	6
Squash, winter	1 c	6
40% Bran cereal, Post	⅔ c	5
Cracklin' Bran cereal	⅔ c	5
Grape-nuts cereal	⅓ c	5
Kellogg's Most cereal	⅔ c	5
Apple, medium	1	5

Food	Serving size	Fiber, grams
Brazil nuts	⅓ c	5
Carrots	1 c	5
Eggplant, boiled	1 c	5
Kale	1 c	5
Squash, summer	1 c	5

Values for vegetables and beans refer to food as cooked.

Sodium Winners

Don't despair: everything you like is not high in sodium.
Here's proof! The foods listed after each category are rea-
sonably low in sodium.

Foods	Range, mg
Beans, Cooked: any unsalted beans and tofu (bean curd)	2–14
Beef, Fresh: most cuts	53–87
Breads: special low-sodium breads	?
Cakes, Prepared: fruitcake	29
Candy: most types	1–75
Cereals, Cold: 100% Natural, Frosted Mini-wheats, puffed rice, puffed wheat, shredded wheat	1–40
Cereals, Hot, Prepared: noninstant only—farina, grits, oatmeal, cream of wheat	1–10
Cheeses: dry curd cottage cheese, natural Swiss	17–74
Chicken, Fresh: most cuts	56–85
Condiments: apple butter, bitters, imitation catsup, garlic clove	0–9
also: horseradish, mayonnaise, Miracle Whip	50–80
Cookies (approx. 1 oz): sugar wafers, macaroons	14–50
Cornish Hen, Duck & Goose: duck or goose, with or w/o skin	58–86

Foods	Range, mg
Crackers (approx. 1 oz): Melba toast, zweiback	1–80
Creams and Creamers: whipped toppings, half & half, imitation coffee whiteners	4–29
Eggs: egg white or whole egg	50–59
Fast Food Vegetables: Burger Chef French fries	33
Fats and Oils: vegetable oil, any type	0
Fish and Shellfish: tuna, low-sodium, canned in water	46
Flour: white, whole wheat, wheat-rye blend	3–4
Frozen Desserts: Creamsicle, Fudgsicle, Popsicle	9–37
Fruit, Canned: if plain—applesauce, apricot, cherries, pears, peaches, pineapple, plum	5–27
Fruit, Dried: apple, apricot, peach, pear, prune, raisins	2–18
Fruit, Frozen: mixed, raspberries, strawberries	3–8
Fruit, Raw: most varieties	0–10
also: cantaloupe, honeydew, mango, plantain	12–24
Gelatin: D-Zerta, all flavors	9
Grains: barley	9–12
Juices, Canned or Bottled: apple, apricot, cranberry cocktail, grape, grapefruit, orange, pineapple, prune	5–9
Juices, Fresh: lemon, lime, orange	2
Juices, from Frozen: most varieties	1–20
Lamb: leg, loin chop, rib chop, shoulder roast	56–77
Milk, Flavored: Nestlé's cocoa mix	30
Miscellaneous: cocoa, jam, jelly, vinegar, yeast	0–2
Nuts and Coconut: almonds, brazil nuts, cashews, chestnuts, coconut, filberts, pecans, walnuts	0–7
Pasta: egg noodles or macaroni, unsalted	1–2
Pork, Fresh: loin chop or roast	68–82
Puddings and Custards: D-Zerta, chocolate	80
Rice and Rice Dishes: instant, white long-grain, or converted	2–6
Seeds: sunflower	11

Foods	Range, mg
Snacks: unsalted popcorn or unsalted pretzels	2–30
also: Nature Valley granola bars	65–80
Soups, Prepared As Directed: many low-sodium varieties	35–75
Sugars: granulated	0
Syrups: corn syrup, chocolate syrup, Kraft dessert toppings, honey	1–20
Turkey, Fresh: light meat or light and dark with skin	59–79
Veal: Cubes, cutlet, loin or rib chops, rump roast	56–83
Vegetables, Canned: LaChoy bamboo shoots or water chestnuts	5–7
Vegetables, Fresh, Cooked: many if unseasoned	1–73
Vegetables, Frozen, Cooked: if plain— asparagus, broccoli, Brussels sprouts, cauliflower, kale, yellow corn	1–82
Vegetables, Raw: cabbage, carrots, celery, cucumber, lettuce, mushrooms, onions, spinach, tomato	2–52

Values for vegetables and beans refer to the food as cooked, except for those listed under "vegetables, Raw" category.

This chart is not designed for people on strict sodium-restricted diets, some of whom may need to avoid some of the foods listed in the chart above.

Sodium Losers

In their natural state, most foods have less than 100 milligrams of sodium per serving. Sadly, their processed counterparts often pack in far more.

Food	Sodium, mg
Bean dishes, canned	980–1200
Beef, corned hash	1520

Food	Sodium, mg
Beef, dried chipped	2472
Borscht	897–985
Bread crumbs, dry	736
Breakfast, fast food	804–1670
Breakfasts, frozen, Hungry-Man	730–1305
Chili, Wendy's	1065
Chili, w or w/o beans, canned	875–1005
Chow mein, canned	835–1675
Corn Dogs, Oscar Mayer	1252
Cottage cheese	849–914
Entrees, frozen	700–1680
Fish & seafood items, frozen, Mrs Paul's	735–2160
Flour: Bisquick, Masa Trigo, or self-rising	885–1520
Fritters, Mrs Paul's	1080–1520
Grits, instant w/imitation ham, Quaker	895
Ham roast, trimmed	1485
Hamburger Helper, prepared	910–1230
Lean 'n Tasty, Oscar Mayer	808–880
Luncheon meats, pork	716–1482
Meat tenderizer, French's	1760
Pancakes, mix or frozen batter	725–1110
Pasta entrees, canned or frozen	720–1233
Pickle, dill	928
Pizza, fast food	800–1500
Pizza, frozen or mix	805–1225
Pretzel twists, hard	1010
Rice, flavored mixes	720–1225
Roll, submarine	783
Salt & flavored salts (1 tsp)	1125–2132
Sandwiches, fast food, many	735–1848
Sardines, oil-pack	735
Seasonings, French's	765–1410
Shrimp, canned	2607
Soups: Cup-a-soup or bouillon cube	698–1066
Soups: canned, regular	760–1125
Soups: chunky-style	1130–1300

Food	Sodium, mg
Soups: wonton, La Choy	2027
Soy sauce	975
TV dinners	925–2190
Teriyaki sauce, from mix, French's	2360
Tomato juice	878
Tomato sauces: plain, barbecue, spaghetti, pizza	700–1240
Tuna Helper, prepared	705–1020
Veal scallopini	918
Vegetables, canned, some	700–1554
Vegetables, frozen, combinations or w/sauce	750–1450

Great Sources of Potassium

All of these foods are not perfect in every way, but each one is very rich in potassium.

Food	Serving Size	Potassium, mg
Peaches, dried	1 c	1520
Avocado	1	1303
Apricots, dried	1 c	1273
Lima beans	1 c	1163
Nonfat dry milk powder	1 c	1160
Veal rump roast, trimmed	4 oz	1158
Dates, chopped	1 c	1153
Sweetened condensed milk	1 c	1136
Raisins	1 c	1106
Pears, dried	1 c	1031
Plaintain	1	1012
Soybeans, cooked	1 c	972
Squash, winter	1 c	945
Evaporated skim milk	1 c	845
Evaporated low-fat milk, Carnation	1 c	832
Navy beans	1 c	790

Food	Serving Size	Potassium, mg
Potato, baked	1	782
Evaporated whole milk	1 c	764
Chocolate shake, Burger Chef	1	762
Whopper sandwich, double	1	760
Great northern beans	1 c	749
Instant breakfast, coffee, Carnation	1 c	736
Apples, dried	1 c	730
Whopper sandwich, double w/cheese	1	730
French fries, homemade	3 oz	726
Peas & potatoes w/cream sauce, Birds Eye	1 c	705
Egg & sausage, Burger Chef	1 pr	688
Spinach	1 c	683
Cantaloupe	½	682
Kidney beans, canned	1 c	673
Brussels sprouts w/cheese sauce, Birds Eye	1 c	670
Sardines, oil-pack	4 oz	669
Flounder, baked w/butter	4 oz	664
Milkshake, Hardee's	1	652
Veal rib chop, trimmed	4 oz	643
Instant breakfast, eggnog, Carnation	1 c	636
Vanilla shake, Burger Chef	1	622
Fun meal, Burger Chef	1 pr	615
Apricots w/syrup, canned	1 c	604
Prune juice	1 c	602
Big Deluxe sandwich, Hardee's	1	594
Peas, split	1 c	592
Whopper w/cheese	1	590
Pumpkin, canned	1 c	588
Parsnips	1 c	587
Molasses, blackstrap	1 tb	585
Spinach	1 c	583
Yogurt, nonfat, plain	1 c	579
Egg & bacon, Burger Chef	1 pr	574
Black-eye peas	1 c	573

Food	Serving Size	Potassium, mg
Veal rump roast, untrimmed	4 oz	562
Nestlé's Quik, chocolate, made w/skim milk	1 c	560
Potato, boiled	1	556
French fries, from frozen	3 oz	555
Tomato juice	1 c	552
Rhubarb, cooked w/sugar	1 c	548
Potato, mashed w/milk	1 c	548
Scallops, steamed	4 oz	540
Veal loin chop, trimmed	4 oz	539
Tomato sauce, Contadina	½ c	537
Yogurt, lowfat, plain	1 c	531
Veal rib chop, untrimmed	4 oz	529
Nestlé's Quik, chocolate, made w/whole milk	1 c	525
Tomato purée, Contadina	½ c	524
Tomatoes, canned	1 c	523
Whopper sandwich	1	520
Dates	10	518
Turkey, light & dark meat w/o skin, chopped	1 c	514
Spinach, canned	1 c	513
Calf liver, fried	4 oz	513
Sweet potato, mashed	1	510
Ratatouille, 10 oz, Stouffers	½	506
Salmon, broiled	4 oz	504
Orange juice, from frozen	1 c	503
Tomatoes, baby, sliced, Contadina	1 c	500
Mixed vegetables w/onion sauce, Birds Eye	1 c	500

Values for beans and vegetables refer to the food as cooked.

Protein, Protein, Everywhere

Among Americans who have enough to eat, rare is the individual who gets too little protein. The animal foods we eat regularly provide so much protein that many Americans take in two to four times their actual need. Here are the top 100 sources, excluding fast foods. Keep in mind that the Recommended Dietary Allowances for adult men and women are 56 and 44 grams per day, respectively.

Food	Serving Size	Protein, grams
Turkey, light & dark meat w/o skin, chopped	1 c	44
Fried chicken TV dinner, Hungry-Man	1	43
Veal loin chop, trimmed	4 oz	39
Veal rib chop, trimmed	4 oz	39
Sliced beef TV dinner, Hungry-Man	1	38
Turkey, light meat w/o skin	4 oz	37
Turkey TV dinner, Hungry-Man	1	37
Beef sirloin steak, trimmed	4 oz	36
Beef round steak, trimmed	4 oz	35
Chicken broiler, light meat w/o skin	4 oz	35
Turkey, dark meat w/o skin	4 oz	35
Veal parmigiana TV dinner, Hungry-Man	1	35
Veal rump roast, trimmed	4 oz	35
Beef round roast, trimmed	4 oz	34
Flounder, baked w/butter	4 oz	34
Pork loin chop, trimmed	4 oz	34
Salisbury steak TV dinner, Hungry-Man	1	34
Veal rump roast, untrimmed	4 oz	34
Beef round roast, untrimmed	4 oz	33
Chicken broiler, light meat w/skin	4 oz	33
Capons, roasted w/skin	4 oz	33
Goose, roasted w/o skin	4 oz	33
Pork roast, trimmed	4 oz	33
Turkey, light & dark meat, w/o skin	4 oz	33
Calf liver, fried	4 oz	33

Food	Serving Size	Protein, grams
Beef round steak, untrimmed	4 oz	32
Cod, broiled w/butter	4 oz	32
Tuna, canned water-pack	4 oz	32
Tuna, oil-pack	4 oz	32
Leg of lamb, trimmed	4 oz	32
Lamb loin chop, broiled, trimmed	4 oz	32
Lamb rib chop, trimmed	4 oz	32
Veal cubes, untrimmed	4 oz	32
Ground round (beef)	4 oz	31
Beef rib roast, trimmed	4 oz	31
Cottage cheese, lowfat 2% fat	1 c	31
Chicken broiler, dark meat w/o skin	4 oz	31
Chicken roaster, light meat w/o skin	4 oz	31
Salmon, broiled	4 oz	31
Veal cutlet, broiled	4 oz	31
Veal rib chop, untrimmed	4 oz	31
Veal rib roast, untrimmed	4 oz	31
Lamb shoulder roast, trimmed	4 oz	30
Fish 'n' chips TV dinner, Hungry-Man	1	30
Beef liver, fried	4 oz	29
Chicken broiler, dark meat w/skin	4 oz	29
Goose, roasted w/skin	4 oz	29
Bluefish, baked w/butter	4 oz	29
Leg of lamb, untrimmed	4 oz	29
Fried chicken TV dinner, Swanson	1	29
Cottage cheese, large curd, 4% fat	1 c	28
Ricotta cheese, part-skim	1 c	28
Ricotta cheese, whole-milk	1 c	28
Chicken roaster, light & dark, w/o skin	4 oz	28
Cornish hen, w/skin	4 oz	28
Shrimp, canned	4 oz	28
Pork loin chop, untrimmed	4 oz	28
Pork roast, untrimmed	4 oz	28
Ground beef, regular	4 oz	27
Beef sirloin steak, untrimmed	4 oz	27
Chicken liver, simmered	4 oz	27

Food	Serving Size	Protein, grams
Chicken roaster, light & dark, w/skin	4 oz	27
Duck, roasted w/o skin	4 oz	27
Cod, canned	1 c	27
Crabmeat, cooked	1 c	27
Lobster, cooked	1 c	27
Sardines, oil-pack	4 oz	27
Cottage cheese, small curd 4%	1 c	26
Chicken breast, fried	½	26
Chicken roaster, dark meat w/o skin	4 oz	26
Scallops, steamed	4 oz	26
Shad, baked w/butter	4 oz	26
Veal loin chop, untrimmed	4 oz	26
Cottage cheese, dry	1 c	25
Cod, broiled w/o fats	4 oz	25
Mackerel, broiled w/butter	4 oz	25
Veal loin chop, broiled, untrimmed	4 oz	25
Crabmeat, canned	1 c	24
Mackerel, canned	4 oz	24
Salmon, smoked	4 oz	24
Sole, baked w/o fats	4 oz	24
Whitefish, smoked	4 oz	24
Lamb shoulder roast, untrimmed	4 oz	24
Sweetened condensed milk	1 c	24
Nonfat dry milk powder	1 c	24
Ham roast, untrimmed	4 oz	24
Lasagne w/meat TV dinner, Hungry-Man	1	24
Beef rib roast, untrimmed	4 oz	23
Haddock, breaded, fried	4 oz	23
Salmon, pink, canned	4 oz	23
Salmon, red, canned	4 oz	23
Rib chop, untrimmed	4 oz	23
Duck, roasted w/skin	4 oz	22
Haddock, panfried	4 oz	22
Ham steak Jubilee, Oscar Mayer	2 sl	22
Fish 'n' chips TV dinner, Swanson	1	22

Food	Serving Size	Protein, grams
Veal parmigiana TV dinner, Swanson	1	22
Hamburger Helper, beef romanoff, prepared	1/5	21
Seafood combo 9 oz, Mrs Paul's	1	20
Veal scallopini	4 oz	20

Protein on the Run

Protein is plentiful at fast food restaurants because of the fish, meat, and cheese items that dominate their menus.

Food	Serving Size	Protein, grams
Triple cheeseburger, Wendy's	1	72
Triple hamburger, Wendy's	1	65
Double cheeseburger, Wendy's	1	50
Whopper, double w/cheese	1	50
Double hamburger, Wendy's	1	44
Whopper, double	1	44
Super supreme pizza, thick-crust, Pizza Hut	2 sl	34
Cheeseburger w/bacon supreme, Jack-in-the-Box	1	33
Single cheeseburger, Wendy's	1	33
Jumbo Jack w/cheese	1	32
Whopper w/cheese	1	32
Ham & cheese supreme, Jack-in-the-Box	1	31
Treasure Chest, Long John Silvers	1 pr	30
Quarter Pounder w/cheese, McDonald's	1	30
Super sandwich, Arby's	1	30
Super supreme pizza, thin-crust, Pizza Hut	2 sl	30
Big Deluxe, Hardee's	1	29
Supreme pizza, thick-crust, Pizza Hut	2 sl	29
Chicken supreme, Jack-in-the-Box	1	28
Jumbo Jack sandwich	1	28

Food	Serving Size	Protein, grams
Mushroom burger, Burger Chef	1	28
Roast beef, big, Hardee's	1	28
Chicken Planks, Long John Silvers	4 pc	27
Beef and cheese sandwich, Arby's	1	27
Super Shef	1	27
Pork-mushroom pizza, thick-crust, Pizza Hut	2 sl	27
Egg & sausage breakfast, Burger Chef	1 pr	26
Eggs breakfast, Jack-in-the-Box	1 pr	26
Sunrise w/sausage, Burger Chef	1 pr	26
Big Mac	1	26
Single hamburger, Wendy's	1	26
Whopper	1	26
Pepperoni pizza, thick-crust, Pizza Hut	2 sl	25
Quarter Pounder, McDonald's	1	24
Cheese pizza, thick-crust, Pizza Hut	2 sl	24
Cheeseburger, double, Burger Chef	1	23
Ham & cheese sandwich, Hardee's	1	23
Shakey's special pizza	2 sl	23
Fish w/batter, Long John Silvers	2 pc	22
Peg Legs, Long John Silvers	5 pc	22
Big Shef	1	22
Roast beef sandwich, Arby's	1	22
Beef & onion pizza, Shakey's	2 sl	22
Italian sausage pizza, Shakey's	2 sl	22
Egg & bacon breakfast, Burger Chef	1 pr	21
Roast beef sandwich, Hardee's	1	21
Pork-mushroom pizza, thin-crust, Pizza Hut	2 sl	21
Supreme pizza, thin-crust, Pizza Hut	2 sl	21
Chicken McNuggets	1 pr	20
Club supreme, Jack-in-the-Box	1	20
Fish, big, Hardee's	1	20
Royal Canadian pizza, Shakey's	2 sl	20

Salute to Vegetable Protein

Contrary to common beliefs, plant foods can and do contribute to our protein needs. Listed below are some plant foods that provide very respectable levels of protein—often without the heavy dose of fat that comes with many animal protein foods.

Food	Serving Size	Protein, grams
Soybeans, cooked	1 c	20
Lentils	1 c	16
Lima beans	1 c	16
Peas, split	1 c	16
Kidney beans, canned	1 c	15
Navy beans	1 c	15
Great northern beans	1 c	14
Black-eye peas	1 c	13
Peanuts, salted	⅓ c	12
Peas & potatoes w/cream sauce, Birds Eye	1 c	12
Potato vermicelli, Green Giant	1 c	11
Butter beans, speckled, Green Giant	1 c	10
Pumpkin seeds	¼ c	10
Lima beans w/butter sauce, Green Giant	1 c	10
Brussels sprouts w/cheese sauce, Birds Eye	1 c	10
Peas & pearl onions, Birds Eye	1 c	10
Tofu (bean curd)	4 oz	9
Walnuts, black, chopped	⅓ c	9
Sunflower seeds	¼ c	9
Almonds, chopped	⅓ c	8
Cashews	⅓ c	8
Coconut milk	1 c	8
Peanut butter	2 tb	8
Peas	1 c	8

Food	Serving Size	Protein, grams
Broccoli w/cheese sauce, Birds Eye	1 c	8
Peas w/cream sauce, Birds Eye	1 c	8
Peas, creamed w/bread topping, Green Giant	1 c	8
Brazil nuts	⅓ c	7
Sesame seeds	¼ c	7
Peas, early w/onions, Green Giant	1 c	7
Brussels sprouts	1 c	7
Greens, collard	1 c	7
Mixed vegetables w/onion sauce, Birds Eye	1 c	7
Mixed Chinese vegetables, canned, La Choy	1 c	6
Spinach	1 c	6
Asparagus, cuts	1 c	6
Green beans w/almonds, Birds Eye	1 c	6
Brussels sprouts w/butter sauce, Green Giant	1 c	6
Corn, green beans & pasta, Birds Eye	1 c	6
Mixed vegetables	1 c	6
Pea pods, Chinese, La Choy	6 oz	6
Spinach	1 c	6
Spinach, creamed Green Giant	1 c	6

Values for vegetables and beans refer to the food as cooked.

The Low-Fat Honor Roll

Fat-watchers, take notice! The foods listed after each category below have a mere 3 grams or less of fat per serving. See the complete chart on each food group for serving sizes.

Alcoholic Beverages: beer, distilled spirits, wine

Beans, Cooked: all types without added fat, except soybeans

Beef, Processed: dried, chipped beef

Breads: white, whole wheat, rye, French, and most loaf breads

Cakes, Prepared: angel food, fruitcake

Candy: gumdrops, hard candy, marshmallows, mints, toffee

Cereals, Cold: most, except granolas

Cereals, Hot, Prepared: farina, grits, oatmeal, wheat

Cheeses: dry cottage cheese

Condiments: apple butter, bitters, catsup, horseradish, mustard, pickles, pimento, Worcestershire sauce

Cookies (approx. 1 oz): fig bars, gingersnaps, raisin-fruit biscuits, spiced wafers

Crackers (approx. 1 oz): graham, rye, saltine, water biscuits, zweiback

Creams and Creamers: imitation powdered and imitation liquid coffee whiteners

Eggs: egg white

Ethnic Dishes: some varieties of chow mein, gefilte fish, matzoh, taco shells, whitefish-pike, wonton soup

Fish and Shellfish: clams, cod, crabmeat, lobster, oysters, scallops, shrimp, sole, water-packed tuna—all without added fat

Flour: cake, cornmeal, rye, white, whole wheat

Frostings: Pillsbury white fluffy, Pillsbury decorator cake and cookie

Frozen Desserts: Creamsicle, Fudgsicle, Lite Fruit Stix, Popsicle

Fruit, Canned: applesauce, apricots, cherries, fruit cocktail, cranberry sauce, peaches, pears, pineapple, plums

Fruit, Dried: apples, apricots, figs, peaches, pears, prunes, raisins

Fruit, Frozen: mixed fruit, raspberries, strawberries
Fruit, Raw: any, except avocado
Gelatin: any
Grains: any without added fats
Jams and Jellies: any
Juices, Canned or Bottled: any
Juices, Fresh: any
Juices, from Frozen: any
Meat Substitutes: Morningstar Farms luncheon slices
Milk, Flavored: cocoa mixes, skim milk with powdered
     milk flavorings
Milk, Plain: low-fat 1%, nonfat dry, skim
Miscellaneous: cocoa, cornstarch, vinegar, yeast
Muffins: English and English-type
Nuts and Coconut: chestnuts
Pancakes, Prep (4-inch): Aunt Jemima Complete mix and
     Aunt Jemima regular frozen batter
Pasta: egg noodles and macaroni—without added fats
Pasta Entrees: Chef Boyardee and Franco-American
     spaghetti with tomato sauce and cheese
Pork, Processed: Oscar Mayer cooked ham
Puddings and Custards: D-zerta and packaged pudding
     mixes made with skim milk
Rice and Rice Dishes: any without added fats
Rolls and Croissants: bagels, brown 'n serve, French,
     hamburger, hard, hot dog, Parker House, sourdough
Salad Dressings: many varieties labelled low-calorie
Sauces: barbecue, many dry gravy mixes made with fat-
     skimmed drippings, sweet and sour, tomato sauce
Snacks: chewing gum, fruit roll-ups, some granola clusters,
     popcorn, pretzels
Soft Drinks: most
Soups, Prep. As Directed: many Campbell and Cup-a-Soup
     varieties, excluding cream soups
Stuffings and Croutons: most croutons
Sugars: any
Syrups: dessert toppings without nuts, honey, molasses,
     pancake syrup

Tea and Coffee: any varieties without added whole milk or
cream
Turkey, Processed: breast, ham, pastrami
Veal: trimmed rump roast
Vegetables, Canned: any without added fats
Vegetables, Fresh, Cooked: any without added fats
Vegetables, Frozen, Cooked: any without added fats,
cheese, or cream sauces
Vegetables, Raw: any plain, except olives in quantity and
coconut
Waffles: Aunt Jemima frozen blueberry, buttermilk, or
original; Downyflake Hot 'n Buttery
Yogurt nonfat and some low-fat varieties

Grease by the Tablespoon

Probably no one would think of swallowing a tablespoon
of vegetable oil. Many foods, though, contain as much
grease as a tablespoon of oil—sometimes even more. Here
are some of the worst offenders in each food category.

Foods	Range, grams
Bean Dishes: beans and franks	14
Beef, Fresh: ground beef, beef rib, or untrimmed sirloin	14–44
Beef, Processed: franks, corned beef hash	14–25
Breakfasts, Frozen: French toast, some Hungry-Man breakfasts	14–35
Cakes, Prepared: cheesecake, walnut cake, cream cake	14–17
Cheeses: ricotta cheeses	20–32
Chicken, Fresh: broiler dark meat w/ skin, roaster light & dark with skin	15–18
Cornish Hen, Duck & Goose: any with skin, goose w/o skin	14–25

Foods	Range, grams
Creams and Creamers: light or heavy whipping cream	19–22
Entrées, Frozen: crepes, meat pies, meatballs, soufflés, Welsh rarebit	17–39
Ethnic Dishes: chili, some brands	17–29
Fast Food Breakfast Items: egg or sausage breakfasts	17–40
Fast Food Desserts: cookies or turnovers, some brands	14–24
Fast Food Pizza: varieties with fatty extras— pepperoni, pork, "supreme"	14–26
Fast Food Platters: deep-fat fried chicken and fish	16–34
Fast Food Sandwiches: jumbo burgers, cheese- burgers, some roast beef, ham & cheese, fried fish, hot dog	14–68
Fast Food Shakes: Frosty, Wendy's	16
Fast Food Vegetables: French fries, some brands of onion rings	16–23
Fats and Oils: vegetable oil, any type (1 tablespoon)	14
Fish and Shellfish: mackerel, deep-fat fried fish, buttery fillets	16–26
Flour: Bisquick (1 cup)	16
Frozen Desserts: ice cream, chocolate chip cookie sandwiches, toasted almond bar	14–24
Fruit, Raw: avocado (1)	37
Lamb: untrimmed cuts	21–41
Meat Substitutes: imitation bacon and sausages	14–15
Milk: eggnog, evaporated whole milk, sweetened condensed milk	19–27
Miscellaneous: baking chocolate or chocolate morsels	15
Nuts and Coconut: coconut and all nuts except chestnuts	16–31

Foods	Range, grams
Pasta Entrées: Fettucine Alfredo, some brands of lasagne, macaroni and cheese, ravioli	14–18
Pastry: Danish or éclair	14–19
Pies: most flavors	16–32
Pizza, Frozen: sausage or deluxe varieties	16–32
Pork, Fresh: roast or loin chops	17–32
Pork, Processed: bacon, many luncheon meats, sausages, franks	14–25
Seeds: pumpkin, sesame, sunflower	16–20
Snacks: Corn dogs	20
TV Dinners: many varieties	15–47
Veal: untrimmed cuts	15–41
Vegetables, Frozen, Cooked: varieties with cream or cheese sauces, or in pastry	14–24

Values for beans and vegetables refer to the foods as cooked.

Part II •

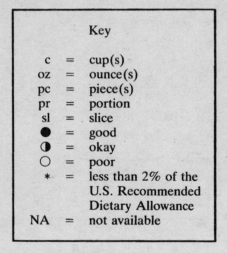

```
              Key

    c   =   cup(s)
    oz  =   ounce(s)
    pc  =   piece(s)
    pr  =   portion
    sl  =   slice
    ●   =   good
    ◑   =   okay
    ○   =   poor
    *   =   less than 2% of the
            U.S. Recommended
            Dietary Allowance
    NA  =   not available
```

Beverages

Alcoholic Beverages

Food	Serving	Calories	Protein g	Fat g	Carbo g	Fiber g	Sodium mg	Potassium mg	Vit A %rda	Vit B1 %rda (thiamin)	Vit B2 %rda (riboflavin)	Vit B3 %rda (niacin)	Vit C %rda	Calcium %rda	Iron %rda
Ale, mild	12 oz	147	2○	0	12●	0	NA	NA	0○	*○	6○	4○	0○	5○	2○
Beer	12 oz	150	1○	0●	14●	0	25●	90○	1○	1○	6○	11●	2○	2○	*○
Beer, lite	12 oz	100	0○	0○	6○	0	NA	NA	NA	NA	NA	NA	NA	NA	NA
Champagne	4 oz	84	0○	0○	3○	0	NA	NA	NA	NA	NA	NA	NA	NA	NA
Gin/rum/whiskey	1 jg	95	0○	0●	0○	0	0●	1○	NA	NA	NA	NA	NA	NA	NA
Wine, dessert	3.5 oz	140	0○	0●	8○	0	4●	77○	NA	1○	1○	NA	1○	1○	NA
Wine, table	3.5 oz	85	0○	0●	4○	0	16●	94○	NA	*○	1○	1○	1○	1○	2○

Juices, Canned or Bottled

Food	Serving	Calories	Protein g	Fat g	Carbo g	Fiber g	Sodium mg	Potassium mg	Vit A %rda	Vit B1 %rda (thiamin)	Vit B2 %rda (riboflavin)	Vit B3 %rda (niacin)	Vit C %rda	Calcium %rda	Iron %rda
Apple	1 c	120	0○	0○	30●	0	5●	250●	1○	3○	1○	3○	2○	2○	8○
Apricot nectar	1 c	145	1○	0●	37●	0	9●	379●	2○	2○	3○	60●	2○	2○	3○

Juices, Canned or Bottled, cont'd.

Food	Serving	Calories	Protein g	Fat g	Carbo g	Fiber g	Sodium mg	Potassium mg	Vit A %rda	Vit B1 %rda (thiamin)	Vit B2 %rda (riboflavin)	Vit B3 %rda (niacin)	Vit C %rda	Calcium %rda	Iron %rda
Cranberry cocktail	1 c	165 ○	0 ●	0 ●	42 ●	0 ○	4 ●	25 ○	* ○	2 ○	2 ○	1 ○	135 ●	1 ○	4 ○
Grape	1 c	165 ○	0 ●	0 ●	42 ●	0 ○	8 ●	293 ●	NA	7 ○	3 ○	3 ○	* ○	3 ○	4 ○
Grapefruit w/sugar	1 c	135 ○	1 ○	0 ●	32 ○	0 ○	3 ●	405 ●	1 ○	5 ○	3 ○	3 ○	130 ●	2 ○	6 ○
Grapefruit, w/o sugar	1 c	100 ○	1 ○	0 ●	24 ○	0 ○	3 ●	400 ●	0 ○	5 ○	3 ○	3 ○	140 ●	2 ○	6 ○
Orange	1 c	120 ○	2 ○	0 ●	28 ●	0 ○	5 ●	496 ●	10 ○	11 ●	3 ○	3 ○	167 ●	3 ○	6 ○
Pineapple w/o sugar	1 c	140 ○	1 ○	0 ●	34 ○	0 ○	5 ●	373 ●	3 ●	9 ○	3 ○	4 ○	133 ●	4 ○	4 ○
Prune	1 c	195 ○	1 ○	0 ●	49 ●	0 ○	5 ●	602 ●	NA	2 ○	2 ○	3 ○	8 ○	4 ○	10 ○
Tomato	1 c	45 ○	2 ○	0 ●	10 ●	0 ○	878 ○	552 ●	39 ●	8 ○	4 ○	10 ●	65 ●	2 ○	12 ●
V-8	6 oz	35 ○	1 ○	0 ●	8 ○	0 ○	640 ○	NA	35 ●	* ○	* ○	4 ○	45 ●	2 ○	4 ○
V-8, low-sodium	6 oz	40 ○	1 ○	0 ●	9 ○	0 ○	60 ●	NA	35 ●	* ○	* ○	4 ○	45 ●	2 ○	4 ○
V-8, spicy-hot	6 oz	40 ○	1 ○	0 ●	8 ○	0 ○	660 ○	NA	35 ●	2 ○	2 ○	4 ○	45 ●	2 ○	4 ○

Juices, Fresh

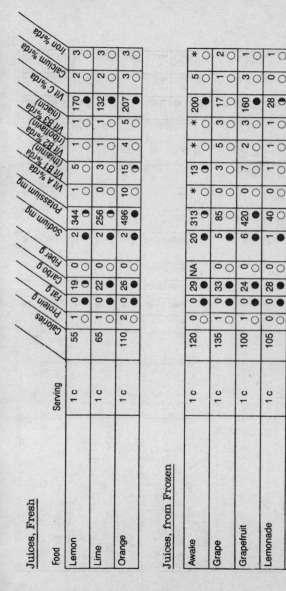

Food	Serving	Calories	Protein g	Fat g	Carbo g	Fiber g	Sodium mg	Potassium mg	Vit A %rda	Vit B1 %rda (thiamin)	Vit B2 %rda (riboflavin)	Vit B3 %rda (niacin)	Vit C %rda	Calcium %rda	Iron %rda
Lemon	1 c	55	1	0	19	0	2	1	1	1	1	1	170	2	3
Lime	1 c	65	1	0	22	0	2	0	3	1	1	1	132	2	3
Orange	1 c	110	2	0	26	0	2	10	15	4	1	5	207	3	3

Juices, from Frozen

Food	Serving	Calories	Protein g	Fat g	Carbo g	Fiber g	Sodium mg	Potassium mg	Vit A %rda	Vit B1 %rda (thiamin)	Vit B2 %rda (riboflavin)	Vit B3 %rda (niacin)	Vit C %rda	Calcium %rda	Iron %rda
Awake	1 c	120	0	0	29	NA	20	*	13	*	*	5	200	*	*
Grape	1 c	135	1	0	33	0	5	0	3	5	3	1	17	2	2
Grapefruit	1 c	100	1	0	24	0	6	0	7	2	3	3	160	1	1
Lemonade	1 c	105	0	0	28	0	1	0	1	*	1	0	28	1	1
Limeade	1 c	100	0	0	27	0	1	*	*	*	*	0	10	*	*

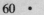

Juices, from Frozen, cont'd.

Food	Serving	Calories	Protein g	Fat g	Carbo g	Fiber g	Sodium mg	Potassium mg	Vit A %rda	Vit B1 %rda (thiamin)	Vit B2 %rda (riboflavin)	Vit B3 %rda (niacin)	Vit C %rda	Calcium %rda	Iron %rda
Orange	1 c	120	2	0	29	0	5	503	11	15	2	5	200	3	1
Orange Plus	1 c	133	0	0	32	NA	12	373	*	13	60	3	200	3	3

Soft Drinks

Food	Serving	Calories	Protein g	Fat g	Carbo g	Fiber g	Sodium mg	Potassium mg	Vit A %rda	Vit B1 %rda (thiamin)	Vit B2 %rda (riboflavin)	Vit B3 %rda (niacin)	Vit C %rda	Calcium %rda	Iron %rda
Club soda	1 c	77	0	0	19	0	39	NA	0	0	0	0	0	NA	NA
Cola	1 c	97	0	0	25	0	16	NA	0	0	0	0	0	NA	NA
Fruit flavors	1 c	113	0	0	30	0	35	NA	0	0	0	0	0	NA	NA
Ginger ale	1 c	77	0	0	19	0	13	0	0	0	0	0	0	NA	NA
Kool-aid, tropical punch	1 c	100	0	0	25	0	1	1	*	*	*	*	15	4	*
Kool-aid, cherry	1 c	90	0	0	23	0	7	1	*	*	*	*	15	4	*
Kool-aid, grape	1 c	90	0	0	23	0	1	1	*	*	*	*	15	4	*

Soft Drinks, cont'd.

Food	Serving	Calories	Protein g	Fat g	Carbo g	Fiber g	Sodium mg	Potassium mg	Vit A %rda	Vit B1 %rda (thiamin)	Vit B2 %rda (riboflavin)	Vit B3 %rda (niacin)	Vit C %rda	Calcium %rda	Iron %rda
Kool-aid, lemonade	1 c	90	0	0	22	0	1	1	*	*	*	*	15	4	*
Lemonade, ready-to-drink Country Time	1 c	90	0	0	23	0	60	7	*	*	*	*	25	*	*
Lemonade, from mix Country Time	1 c	100	0	0	25	0	30	15	*	*	*	*	15	*	*
Root beer	1 c	100	0	0	26	0	NA	0	0	0	0	0	0	NA	NA
Tang, orange	1 c	120	0	0	30	0	2	40	*	*	*	*	200	4	2
Yoo-Hoo	1 c	124	3	1	24	NA	22	9	2	9	9	9	9	9	2

Tea and Coffee

Food	Serving	Calories	Protein g	Fat g	Carbo g	Fiber g	Sodium mg	Potassium mg	Vit A %rda	Vit B1 %rda (thiamin)	Vit B2 %rda (riboflavin)	Vit B3 %rda (niacin)	Vit C %rda	Calcium %rda	Iron %rda
Cafe Francaise General Foods	¾ c	60	1	3	7	0	95	135	*	*	4	*	*	*	*
Cafe Vienna General Foods	¾ c	60	1	2	10	0	95	125	*	*	2	*	*	*	*

Tea and Coffee, cont'd.

Food	Serving	Calories	Protein g	Fat g	Carbo g	Fiber g	Sodium mg	Potassium mg	Vit A %rda	Vit B1 %rda (thiamin)	Vit B2 %rda (riboflavin)	Vit B3 %rda (niacin)	Vit C %rda	Calcium %rda	Iron %rda
Coffee, from instant	¾ c	2	0	0	0	0	2	65	0	0	*	3	0	0	1
Irish mocha mint General Foods	¾ c	50	1	2	7	0	90	135	*	*	*	*	*	*	*
Nestea, lemon	¾ c	2	0	0	0	0	8	60	*	*	*	*	*	*	*
Nestea, sugar/lemon	¾ c	70	0	0	17	0	10	40	*	*	*	*	*	*	*
Orange cappuccino General Foods	¾ c	60	1	2	10	0	100	125	*	*	*	*	*	*	*
Postum	¾ c	12	0	0	3	0	3	100	*	*	*	4	*	*	*
Suisse mocha General Foods	¾ c	60	1	3	7	0	40	120	*	*	*	*	*	*	*

Dairy & Eggs
Cheeses

Food	Serving	Calories	Protein g	Fat g	Carbo g	Fiber g	Sodium mg	Potassium mg	Vit A %rda	Vit B1 %rda (thiamin)	Vit B2 %rda (riboflavin)	Vit B3 %rda (niacin)	Vit C %rda	Calcium %rda	Iron %rda
American	1 oz	105	6	9	0	0	406	46	7	1	6	*	0	17	1
Blue	1 oz	100	6	8	1	0	396	73	4	1	6	2	0	15	1
Camembert, wedge	1	115	8	9	0	0	324	71	7	1	11	1	0	15	1
Cheddar	1 oz	115	7	9	0	0	176	28	6	1	6	*	0	20	1
Cheez Whiz	1 oz	80	5	6	2	0	370	NA	4	*	6	*	0	15	*
Cottage, large curd 4%	1 c	235	28	10	6	0	909	190	7	3	22	2	*	14	2
Cottage, small curd 4%	1 c	220	26	9	6	0	849	177	7	3	20	2	*	13	2
Cottage, dry	1 c	125	25	1	3	0	17	47	1	3	12	1	0	5	2
Cottage, lowfat 2%	1 c	205	31	4	8	0	914	217	3	3	25	2	*	16	2
Cream cheese	2 tb	100	2	10	1	0	84	34	8	*	4	*	0	2	2
Fondue Swiss Knight	1 oz	60	4	5	1	0	185	NA	4	*	6	*	0	15	*

Cheeses, cont'd.

Food	Serving	Calories	Protein g	Fat g	Carbo g	Fiber g	Sodium mg	Potassium mg	Vit A %rda	Vit B1 %rda (thiamin)	Vit B2 %rda (riboflavin)	Vit B3 %rda (niacin)	Vit C %rda	Calcium %rda	Iron %rda
Golden Image, cheddar	1 oz	110	7	9	1	0	170	NA	4	*	6	*	20	*	*
Light'n Lively, American (1.3 sl)	1 oz	70	6	4	2	0	410	NA	4	*	6	*	20	*	*
Mozzarella, part-skim	1 oz	80	8	5	1	0	132	27	4	1	6	0	21	1	1
Mozzarella, whole milk	1 oz	90	6	7	1	0	106	21	5	*	5	0	16	1	1
Parmesan, grated	1 tb	25	2	2	0	0	94	5	1	*	1	0	7	*	*
Provolone	1 oz	100	7	8	1	0	248	39	5	1	5	0	21	1	1
Ricotta, part-skim	1 c	342	28	13	0	0	310	21	21	3	27	1	67	6	6
Ricotta, whole-milk	1 c	432	28	32	0	0	208	24	24	2	28	1	51	5	5
Snack Mate spread, American or cheddar	1 oz	80	5	6	2	0	NA	NA	4	*	8	*	10	*	*
Swiss	1 oz	105	8	8	1	0	74	31	5	1	6	0	27	1	*
Velveeta	1 oz	80	5	6	2	0	430	NA	4	*	6	*	15	*	*

Cheeses, cont'd.

Food	Serving	Calories	Protein g	Fat g	Carbo g	Fiber g	Sodium mg	Potassium mg	Vit A %rda	Vit B1 %rda (thiamin)	Vit B2 %rda (riboflavin)	Vit B3 %rda (niacin)	Vit C %rda	Calcium %rda	Iron %rda
Wispride cheddar	1 oz	90	5 ●	7 ●	2	0	205 ●	110	4	*	8	*	*	35 ●	*
Wispride smoked	1 oz	90	5 ●	6 ●	3	0	235 ●	98	4	*	10 ●	*	*	15 ●	*
Wispride wine	1 oz	100	5	9	1	0	250 ●	75	4	*	8	*	*	15 ●	*

Creams and Creamers

Food	Serving	Calories	Protein g	Fat g	Carbo g	Fiber g	Sodium mg	Potassium mg	Vit A %rda	Vit B1 %rda (thiamin)	Vit B2 %rda (riboflavin)	Vit B3 %rda (niacin)	Vit C %rda	Calcium %rda	Iron %rda
Cool Whip	¼ c	56	0	4	4	0	8 ●	4	NA	*	*	*	*	*	*
Dream Whip	¼ c	32	0	NA	4	0	16 ●	28	NA	*	*	*	*	*	*
Half-and-half	1 tb	20	0	2 ●	1	0	7 ●	19	0	*	1	1	*	2	*
Heavy whipping	¼ c	205	1	22	2	0	19 ●	45	18	1	4	1	1	4	*
Imitation liquid, frozen	1 tb	20	0	1 ●	2	0	12 ●	29	*	0	0	0	0	*	*
Imitation powdered	1 ts	10	0	1 ●	1	0	4 ●	16	*	0	0	0	0	*	*

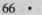

Creams and Creamers, cont'd.

Food	Serving	Calories	Protein g	Fat g	Carbo g	Fiber g	Sodium mg	Potassium mg	Vit A %rda	Vit B1 %rda (thiamin)	Vit B2 %rda (riboflavin)	Vit B3 %rda (niacin)	Vit C %rda	Calcium %rda	Iron %rda
Imitation sour	¼ c	104	2	10	3	0	61	95	0	2	6	*	1	7	*
Imitation whipped, frozen	¼ c	60	*	5	4	0	9	4	3	0	0	0	0	*	*
Light whipping	¼ c	175	1	19	2	0	24	58	14	1	5	*	1	4	*
Sour	¼ c	124	2	12	3	0	29	83	9	1	5	*	1	7	*
Table	1 tb	30	0	3	1	0	6	18	2	*	1	*	*	1	*
Whipped topping D-zerta	¼ c	32	0	4	0	0	28	32	NA	*	*	*	*	*	*
Whipped topping, aerosol	¼ c	39	1	3	2	0	20	22	3	*	1	0	0	2	*

Eggs

Food	Serving	Calories	Protein g	Fat g	Carbo g	Fiber g	Sodium mg	Potassium mg	Vit A %rda	Vit B1 %rda (thiamin)	Vit B2 %rda (riboflavin)	Vit B3 %rda (niacin)	Vit C %rda	Calcium %rda	Iron %rda
Eggstra Tillie Lewis	½ pk	50	5	2	4	0	105	130	*	15	15	*	2	2	5
Fried w/butter	1	85	6	6	1	NA	58	6	2	8	8	*	0	3	5

Eggs, cont'd.

Food	Serving	Calories	Protein g	Fat g	Carbo g	Fiber g	Sodium mg	Potassium mg	Vit A %rda	Vit B1 %rda (thiamin)	Vit B2 %rda (riboflavin)	Vit B3 %rda (niacin)	Vit C %rda	Calcium %rda	Iron %rda
Hard-cooked	1	80	6	6	1	0	61	5	3	3	8	*	0	3	6
Poached	1	80	6	6	1	0	NA	5	3	3	8	*	0	3	6
Scrambled w/milk	1	95	6	7	1	0	NA	6	3	3	9	*	0	5	5
Scramblers	¼ c	64	7	3	3	0	126	NA	33	35	*	*	4	11	11
White, raw	1	15	3	0	0	0	50	45	0	*	5	*	0	0	*
Whole, raw	1	80	6	6	1	0	59	65	3	3	9	*	0	3	6
Yolk, raw	1	65	3	6	0	0	9	15	3	3	4	*	0	3	5

Milk, Flavored

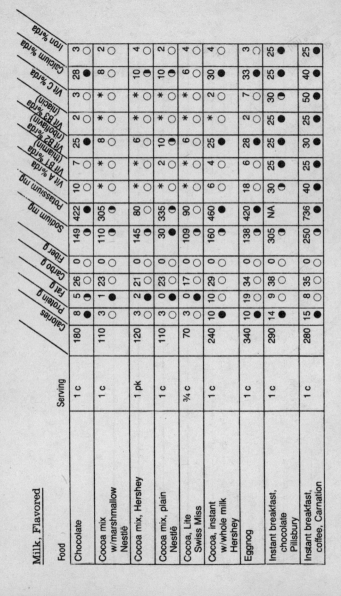

Food	Serving	Calories	Protein g	Fat g	Carbo g	Fiber g	Sodium mg	Potassium mg	Vit A % rda	Vit B1 % rda (thiamin)	Vit B2 % rda (riboflavin)	Vit B3 % rda (niacin)	Vit C % rda	Calcium % rda	Iron % rda
Chocolate	1 c	180	8 ●	5 ●	26 ○	0	149 ○	422 ●	10 ○	7 ○	25 ●	2 ○	3 ○	28 ●	3 ○
Cocoa mix w/marshmallow Nestlé	1 c	110	3 ○	1 ●	23 ○	0	110 ○	305 ●	* ○	* ○	8 ○	* ○	* ○	8 ○	2 ○
Cocoa mix, Hershey	1 pk	120	3 ○	2 ●	21 ○	0	145 ○	80 ○	* ○	6 ○	6 ○	* ○	* ○	10 ●	4 ○
Cocoa mix, plain Nestlé	1 c	110	3 ○	0 ●	23 ○	0	30 ○	335 ●	* ○	2 ○	10 ●	* ○	* ○	10 ●	2 ○
Cocoa, Lite Swiss Miss	¾ c	70	3 ○	0 ●	17 ○	0	109 ○	90 ○	2 ○	6 ○	6 ○	* ○	* ○	6 ○	4 ○
Cocoa, instant w/whole milk Hershey	1 c	240	10 ●	10 ●	29 ○	0	160 ●	460 ●	6 ○	4 ○	25 ●	2 ○	2 ○	30 ●	4 ○
Eggnog	1 c	340	10 ●	19 ○	34 ○	0	138 ●	420 ●	18 ○	6 ○	28 ●	7 ○	7 ○	33 ●	3 ○
Instant breakfast, chocolate Pillsbury	1 c	290	14 ●	9 ○	38 ○	0	305 ●	NA	30 ●	25 ●	25 ●	30 ●	30 ●	25 ●	25 ●
Instant breakfast, coffee, Carnation	1 c	280	15 ●	8 ●	35 ○	0	250 ●	736 ●	40 ●	25 ●	30 ●	50 ●	50 ●	40 ●	25 ●

Milk, Flavored, cont'd.

Food	Serving	Calories	Protein g	Fat g	Carbo g	Fiber g	Sodium mg	Potassium mg	Vit A %rda	Vit B1 %rda (thiamin)	Vit B2 %rda (riboflavin)	Vit B3 %rda (niacin)	Vit C %rda	Calcium %rda	Iron %rda
Instant breakfast, eggnog, Carnation	1 c	280	15	8	34	0	315	636	40	25	30	25	50	40	25
Instant breakfast, strawberry Pillsbury	1 c	290	14	9	39	0	300	NA	30	25	25	25	30	25	25
Instant breakfast, vanilla Pillsbury	1 c	290	14	9	39	0	315	NA	30	25	25	25	30	25	25
Quik, chocolate w/skim milk	1 c	170	9	1	31	0	160	560	10	6	30	*	4	2	2
Quik, chocolate w/whole milk	1 c	240	9	9	30	0	155	525	6	6	25	*	4	2	2
Quik, strawberry w/whole milk	1 c	240	8	8	33	0	120	NA	6	6	25	*	2	*	3
Sweet condensed	1 c	980	24	27	166	0	389	1136	20	19	75	3	13	87	3

Milk, Plain

Food	Serving	Calories	Protein g	Fat g	Carbo g	Fiber g	Sodium mg	Potassium mg	Vit A %rda	Vit B1 %rda (thiamin)	Vit B2 %rda (riboflavin)	Vit B3 %rda (niacin)	Vit C %rda	Calcium %rda	Iron %rda
Buttermilk	1 c	100	8	2	12	0	257	371	2	5	22	1	3	29	1
Evaporated lowfat Carnation	1 c	220	18	6	24	0	276	832	20	4	40	*	*	60	*
Evaporated skim	1 c	200	19	1	29	0	294	845	20	7	46	2	5	74	4
Evaporated whole	1 c	340	17	19	25	0	266	764	12	8	47	3	8	66	3
Lowfat 1%	1 c	105	9	2	12	0	122	397	10	7	25	1	3	31	1
Lowfat 2%	1 c	125	9	5	12	0	150	397	10	7	25	1	3	31	1
Nonfat dry powder	1 c	245	24	0	35	0	373	1160	32	19	70	3	7	84	1
Skim	1 c	85	8	0	12	0	127	406	10	6	20	1	3	30	1
Whole	1 c	150	8	8	11	0	122	370	6	6	24	1	3	29	1

Yogurt

Food	Serving	Calories	Protein g	Fat g	Carbo g	Fiber g	Sodium mg	Potassium mg	Vit A %rda	Vit B1 %rda (thiamin)	Vit B2 %rda (riboflavin)	Vit B3 %rda (niacin)	Vit C %rda	Calcium %rda	Iron %rda
Coffee, lowfat Dannon	1 c	200	11	4	32	0	255	NA	2	4	20	*	*	35	*
Fruit, Colombo	1 c	230	8	6	36	0	148	NA	2	6	20	*	*	20	*
Fruit, lowfat Dannon	1 c	260	10	3	49	0	250	NA	*	2	20	*	*	35	*
Lemon, lowfat Dannon	1 c	200	11	4	32	0	255	NA	2	4	20	*	*	35	*
Lowfat, fruit	1 c	230	10	3	42	0	133	439	2	5	24	1	2	34	1
Lowfat, plain	1 c	145	12	4	16	0	159	531	3	7	29	2	3	42	1
Nonfat, plain	1 c	125	13	0	17	0	174	579	0	7	31	2	3	45	1
Plain, Colombo	1 c	151	9	7	13	0	159	NA	*	15	21	*	3	31	1
Plain, lowfat Dannon	1 c	150	12	4	17	0	235	NA	2	4	30	*	*	40	*
Vanilla, lowfat Dannon	1 c	200	11	4	32	0	255	NA	2	4	20	*	*	35	*
Whole milk, plain	1 c	140	8	7	11	0	105	351	6	5	19	1	2	27	1

Yogurt, cont'd.

Food	Serving	Calories	Protein g	Fat g	Carbo g	Fiber g	Sodium mg	Potassium mg	Vit A %rda	Vit B1 %rda (thiamin)	Vit B2 %rda (riboflavin)	Vit B3 %rda (niacin)	Vit C %rda	Calcium %rda	Iron %rda
Yoplait, custard style, fruit flavors	1	180	7	4	30	0	105	NA	2	4	20	*	25	*	*
Yoplait, custard style, plain w/honey	1	160	7	4	23	0	110	NA	2	4	20	*	25	*	*
Yoplait, custard style, vanilla	1	180	7	4	30	0	110	NA	2	4	20	*	25	*	*

Fruits, Vegetables, Nuts & Seeds

Bean Dishes

Food	Serving	Calories	Protein g	Fat g	Carbo g	Fiber g	Sodium mg	Potassium mg	Vit A % rda	Vit B1 % rda (thiamin)	Vit B2 % rda (riboflavin)	Vit B3 % rda (niacin)	Vit C % rda	Calcium % rda	Iron % rda
Bean salad, canned Green Giant	1 c	190	4	1	42	NA	NA	6	8	6	2	20	6	6	10
Beans & franks, 7.9-oz cn, Campbell	1	350	14	14	42	NA	1200	4	4	4	8	8	10	10	20
Homestyle beans, 7.9-oz cn, Campbell	1	270	11	4	48	NA	1200	2	4	2	4	6	10	10	20
Pork & beans 8-oz can, Campbell	1	250	11	4	44	NA	980	2	4	*	2	4	10	10	15

Beans, Cooked

Food	Serving	Calories	Protein g	Fat g	Carbo g	Fiber g	Sodium mg	Potassium mg	Vit A % rda	Vit B1 % rda (thiamin)	Vit B2 % rda (riboflavin)	Vit B3 % rda (niacin)	Vit C % rda	Calcium % rda	Iron % rda
Bean sprouts La Choy	1 c	23	3	0	2	NA	161	NA	NA	NA	NA	NA	NA	NA	NA
Bean sprouts, mung, cooked	1 c	35	4	0	7	4	5	195	1	7	8	5	13	2	6
Bean sprouts, mung, raw	1 c	35	4	0	7	2	5	234	0	0	9	8	33	2	8
Black-eye peas	1 c	190	13	1	35	NA	14	573	1	27	6	5	NA	4	18

Beans, Cooked, cont'd.

Food	Serving	Calories	Protein g	Fat g	Carbo g	Fiber g	Sodium mg	Potassium mg	Vit A %rda	Vit B1 %rda (thiamin)	Vit B2 %rda (riboflavin)	Vit B3 %rda (niacin)	Vit C %rda	Calcium %rda	Iron %rda
Butter beans, speckled Green Giant	1 c	280	10	11	34	NA	NA	NA	*	70	4	*	6	4	10
Great northern	1 c	210	14	1	38	16	5	749	0	17	8	7	0	9	27
Kidney, canned	1 c	230	15	1	42	19	844	673	0	9	6	8	NA	7	26
Lentils	1 c	210	16	0	39	7	4	498	1	9	7	6	0	5	23
Lima	1 c	260	16	1	49	18	2	1163	NA	17	6	7	NA	6	33
Navy	1 c	225	15	1	40	17	2	790	0	18	8	7	0	10	28
Peas, split	1 c	230	16	1	42	NA	4	592	2	20	11	9	NA	2	19
Soybeans, cooked	1 c	234	20	10	19	NA	4	972	1	25	9	6	0	13	27
Tofu (bean curd)	4 oz	82	9	5	3	NA	8	48	0	5	2	1	0	15	12

Fruit, Canned

Food	Serving	Calories	Protein g	Fat g	Carbo g	Fiber g	Sodium mg	Potassium mg	Vit A %rda	Vit B1 %rda (thiamin)	Vit B2 %rda (riboflavin)	Vit B3 %rda (niacin)	Vit C %rda	Calcium %rda	Iron %rda
Applesauce w/o sugar	1 c	100	0 ○	0 ○	26	NA	5 ●	190	2 ○	3 ○	1 ○	3 ○	1 ○	1 ○	7 ○
Applesauce w/sugar	1 c	230	1 ○	0 ●	61	NA	5 ●	166	2 ○	3 ○	1 ○	5 ○	1 ○	1 ○	7 ○
Apricots w/syrup	1 c	220	2 ○	0 ●	57 ○	NA	27 ●	604 ●	90 ●	3 ○	5 ○	17 ○	3 ○	3 ○	4 ○
Cherries, sour	1 c	105	2 ○	0 ●	26	3 ●	9 ●	317 ●	33 ●	5 ○	3 ○	20 ●	4 ○	4 ○	4 ○
Cocktail w/syrup	1 c	195	1 ○	0 ●	50	NA	13 ●	411 ●	7 ○	3 ○	2 ○	8 ○	2 ○	2 ○	6 ○
Cranberry sauce	1 c	405	0 ○	1 ●	104	NA	75 ●	83 ○	1 ○	2 ○	2 ○	10 ○	2 ○	3 ○	3 ○
Peach slices w/syrup	1 c	200	1 ○	0 ●	51	NA	15 ●	333 ●	22 ●	2 ○	3 ○	13 ○	4 ○	1 ○	4 ○
Peach slices, juice-pack	1 c	75	1 ○	0 ●	20 ●	NA	5 ●	334 ●	22 ●	1 ○	4 ○	12 ○	4 ○	1 ○	4 ○
Pears w/syrup	1 c	195	1 ○	1 ●	50	NA	15 ●	214 ●	0 ○	2 ○	3 ○	5 ○	1 ○	1 ○	3 ○
Pineapple chunks w/syrup	1 c	190	1 ○	0 ●	49	NA	7 ●	245 ●	3 ○	13 ●	3 ○	30 ●	3 ○	3 ○	4 ○
Plum w/syrup	1 c	215	1 ○	0 ○	56	NA	10 ●	367 ●	63 ●	3 ○	5 ○	8 ○	2 ○	13 ●	13 ●

Fruit, Dried

Food	Serving	Calories	Protein g	Fat g	Carbo g	Fiber g	Sodium mg	Potassium mg	Vit A % rda	Vit B1 % rda (thiamin)	Vit B2 % rda (riboflavin)	Vit B3 % rda (niacin)	Vit C % rda	Calcium % rda	Iron % rda
Apples	1 c	353	1	2	92	NA	7	730	NA	*	4	3	17	4	11
Apricots	1 c	340	7	1	86	NA	12	1273	283	1	12	22	27	9	40
Fig, medium	1	40	1	0	10	9	1	97	1	2	2	1	2	2	2
Peaches	1 c	420	5	1	109	NA	10	1520	125	1	18	43	48	8	53
Pears	1 c	482	6	3	121	NA	13	1031	3	1	19	6	22	6	13
Prunes	5	110	1	0	29	8	2	298	14	3	4	4	2	2	9
Raisins	1 c	420	4	0	112	10	18	1106	1	11	7	4	2	9	28

Fruit, Frozen

Food	Serving	Calories	Protein g	Fat g	Carbo g	Fiber g	Sodium mg	Potassium mg	Vit A %rda	Vit B1 %rda (thiamin)	Vit B2 %rda (riboflavin)	Vit B3 %rda (niacin)	Vit C %rda	Calcium %rda	Iron %rda
Mixed fruit Birds Eye	1 c	280	2	0	72	NA	8	370	16	*	8	4	90	*	4
Raspberries w/sugar	1 c	318	2	1	79	NA	3	322	5	5	11	10	113	5	10
Strawberries, sweetened	10 oz	310	1	1	79	NA	6	318	2	4	10	7	252	4	11

Fruit, Raw

Food	Serving	Calories	Protein g	Fat g	Carbo g	Fiber g	Sodium mg	Potassium mg	Vit A %rda	Vit B1 %rda (thiamin)	Vit B2 %rda (riboflavin)	Vit B3 %rda (niacin)	Vit C %rda	Calcium %rda	Iron %rda
Apple, large	1	125	0	1	31	7	2	233	4	2	2	1	13	3	3
Apple, medium	1	80	0	1	20	5	2	152	2	1	2	1	10	2	2
Apricots	3	55	1	0	14	2	0	301	58	2	2	3	18	2	3
Avocado	1	370	5	37	13	4	22	1303	16	16	25	18	50	7	7
Banana, medium	1	100	1	0	26	2	2	440	4	4	4	4	20	1	4
Blackberries	1 c	85	2	1	19	7	1	245	6	3	4	3	50	5	7

Fruit, Raw, cont'd.

Food	Serving	Calories	Protein g	Fat g	Carbo g	Fiber g	Sodium mg	Potassium mg	Vit A %rda	Vit B1 %rda (thiamin)	Vit B2 %rda (riboflavin)	Vit B3 %rda (niacin)	Vit C %rda	Calcium %rda	Iron %rda
Blueberries	1 c	90	1	1	22	NA	1	117	3	3	5	4	33	2	8
Cantaloupe	½	80	2	0	20	3	24	682	185	7	5	8	150	4	6
Cherries, sweet	10	45	1	0	12	1	0	129	1	2	2	2	12	2	2
Cranberries	1 c	44	0	0	10	4	2	78	1	2	1	1	17	1	3
Dates	10	220	2	0	58	7	1	518	1	5	5	9	0	5	13
Dates, chopped	1 c	490	4	1	130	16	2	1153	2	11	11	20	0	11	29
Grapefruit	½	50	1	0	13	2	1	166	11	3	1	1	73	2	3
Grapes, seedless	10	35	0	0	9	0	1	87	1	2	1	1	3	1	1
Honeydew	1/10	50	1	0	11	1	14	374	1	4	2	5	57	2	3
Lemon	1	20	1	0	6	NA	1	102	0	2	1	1	65	2	2
Mango	1 c	109	1	1	28	NA	12	312	158	5	5	9	97	2	4

Fruit, Raw, cont'd.

Food	Serving	Calories	Protein g	Fat g	Carbo g	Fiber g	Sodium mg	Potassium mg	Vit A % rda	Vit B1 % rda (thiamin)	Vit B2 % rda (riboflavin)	Vit B3 % rda (niacin)	Vit C % rda	Calcium % rda	Iron % rda
Nectarine	1	88	1○	0●	24●	3●	8●	406●	46●	NA	NA	NA	30●	1○	4○
Orange	1	65	1○	0●	16●	3●	1●	263○	5○	9●	3○	3○	110●	5○	3○
Orange, chopped	1 c	90	2○	0●	22●	4●	2●	360●	7○	12●	4○	4○	150●	7○	4○
Papaya	1 c	55	1○	0●	14●	NA	3●	328●	49●	4○	4○	2○	130●	3○	2○
Peach	1	40	1○	0●	10○	1○	1●	202●	27●	1○	3○	5○	12○	1○	3○
Pear	1	100	1○	1●	25●	4●	0●	213●	1○	2○	4○	1○	12○	1○	3○
Pineapple	1 c	80	1○	0●	21●	2○	1●	226●	2○	9○	3○	2○	43●	1○	3○
Plantain	1	313	3○	1●	82●	NA	13●	1012●	NA	11●	6○	8○	62●	2○	10●
Plum	1	30	0○	0●	8○	1○	1●	112○	3○	1○	1○	2○	7○	3○	2○
Pomegranate	1	97	1●	1●	25	NA	5●	399●	*○	3○	3○	3○	10○	1○	3○
Raspberries	1 c	70	1○	1●	17●	9●	1●	207●	3○	3○	6○	6○	52●	3○	6○

Fruit, Raw, cont'd.

Food	Serving	Calories	Protein g	Fat g	Carbo g	Fiber g	Sodium mg	Potassium mg	Vit A %rda	Vit B1 %rda (thiamin)	Vit B2 %rda (riboflavin)	Vit B3 %rda (niacin)	Vit C %rda	Calcium %rda	Iron %rda
Rhubarb, cooked w/sugar	1 c	380	1	0	97	NA	5	548	4	3	8	4	27	9	21
Strawberries	1 c	55	1	1	13	3	2	244	2	3	6	5	147	8	3
Tangerine	1	40	1	0	10	2	1	108	7	3	1	1	45	2	3
Watermelon	1/16	110	2	1	27	4	8	426	50	9	8	5	50	12	3

Nuts and Coconut

Food	Serving	Calories	Protein g	Fat g	Carbo g	Fiber g	Sodium mg	Potassium mg	Vit A %rda	Vit B1 %rda (thiamin)	Vit B2 %rda (riboflavin)	Vit B3 %rda (niacin)	Vit C %rda	Calcium %rda	Iron %rda
Almonds, chopped	1/3 c	258	8	23	8	6	1	335	0	7	24	8	*	11	10
Brazil	1/3 c	305	7	31	5	5	0	334	*	30	3	5	NA	10	8
Cashews	1/3 c	262	8	21	14	NA	7	217	1	13	7	4	NA	10	2
Chestnuts, shelled	1/3 c	103	2	1	22	4	3	242	NA	8	7	2	NA	5	1
Coconut milk	1 c	605	8	60	13	0	NA	NA	0	5	*	10	8	21	4

Nuts and Coconut, cont'd.

Food	Serving	Calories	Protein g	Fat g	Carbo g	Fiber g	Sodium mg	Potassium mg	Vit A %rda	Vit B1 %rda (thiamin)	Vit B2 %rda (riboflavin)	Vit B3 %rda (niacin)	Vit C %rda	Calcium %rda	Iron %rda
Coconut, shredded	1/3 c	92 ○	1 ○	9 ●	3 ○	NA	6 ●	68 ○	0 ○	1 ○	* ○	1 ○	1 ○	* ○	3 ○
Filberts, chopped	1/3 c	243 ○	5 ○	24 ○	6 ○	NA	1 ●	270 ●	NA	12 ●	NA	2 ○	* ○	8 ○	7 ○
Peanut butter	2 tb	190 ●	8 ●	16 ○	6 ○	2 ○	162 ●	200 ●	NA	2 ○	2 ○	24 ●	0 ○	2 ○	4 ○
Peanuts, salted	1/3 c	280 ●	12 ●	24 ○	9 ●	4 ●	200 ●	324 ●	NA	10 ●	4 ○	41 ●	0 ○	4 ○	6 ○
Pecans, chopped	1/3 c	270 ●	4 ●	28 ○	6 ○	3 ●	1 ●	237 ●	1 ○	22 ●	3 ○	2 ○	1 ○	3 ○	5 ○
Walnuts, black, chopped	1/3 c	262 ●	9 ●	25 ○	6 ○	2 ○	1 ●	192 ○	3 ○	6 ○	3 ○	2 ○	NA	* ○	14 ●

Seeds

Food	Serving	Calories	Protein g	Fat g	Carbo g	Fiber g	Sodium mg	Potassium mg	Vit A %rda	Vit B1 %rda (thiamin)	Vit B2 %rda (riboflavin)	Vit B3 %rda (niacin)	Vit C %rda	Calcium %rda	Iron %rda
Pumpkin	1/4 c	194 ●	10 ●	16 ○	5 ○	NA	NA	347 ●	1 ○	6 ○	4 ○	4 ○	NA	2 ○	22 ●
Sesame	1/4 c	218 ●	7 ●	20 ●	7 ○	NA	NA	NA	NA	5 ○	3 ○	10 ○	0 ○	4 ○	5 ○
Sunflower	1/4 c	203 ●	9 ●	17 ●	7 ○	NA	11 ●	334 ●	* ○	47 ●	5 ○	10 ○	NA	4 ○	14 ●

Vegetables, Canned

Food	Serving	Calories	Protein g	Fat g	Carbo g	Fiber g	Sodium mg	Potassium mg	Vit A %rda	Vit B1 %rda (thiamin)	Vit B2 %rda (riboflavin)	Vit B3 %rda (niacin)	Vit C %rda	Calcium %rda	Iron %rda
Asparagus spears Green Giant	1 c	40	3	1	5	NA	440	NA	15	4	6	6	60	2	2
Bamboo shoots La Choy	1 c	23	2	0	4	NA	5	NA	NA	NA	NA	NA	NA	NA	NA
Beans, green	1 c	30	2	0	7	4	338	128	13	3	4	2	8	6	11
Beans, wax	1 c	30	2	0	7	NA	564	128	3	3	4	2	12	6	11
Beets, sliced	1 c	65	2	0	15	4	479	284	1	1	3	1	8	3	7
Carrots	1 c	45	1	0	10	5	386	186	465	2	3	3	5	5	6
Chop suey vegetables, La Choy	1 c	53	3	0	10	NA	1339	NA	NA	NA	NA	NA	NA	NA	NA
Corn, white Green Giant	1 c	150	4	1	30	NA	310	NA	*	2	6	6	25	*	4
Corn, yellow, creamed	1 c	210	5	2	51	NA	671	248	17	5	8	13	22	1	8
Corn, yellow, plain	1 c	175	5	1	43	10	488	204	15	4	8	12	18	1	6
Mexicorn Green Giant	1 c	150	4	1	30	NA	520	NA	6	2	6	6	25	*	4

Vegetables, Canned, cont'd.

Food	Serving	Calories	Protein g	Fat g	Carbo g	Fiber g	Sodium mg	Potassium mg	Vit A %rda	Vit B1 %rda (thiamin)	Vit B2 %rda (riboflavin)	Vit B3 %rda (niacin)	Vit C %rda	Calcium %rda	Iron %rda
Mixed Chinese La Choy	1 c	35	6	0	2	NA	144	NA	NA	NA	NA	NA	NA	NA	NA
Mushrooms, whole or pieces, Green Giant	2 oz	14	1	0	2	NA	155	NA	*	*	2	2	*	*	*
Peas	1 c	150	8	1	29	13	493	163	23	10	7	7	23	4	18
Peas, early w/onions Green Giant	1 c	120	7	1	22	NA	700	NA	15	6	4	4	35	2	10
Pumpkin	1 c	80	2	1	19	NA	12	588	314	5	7	8	20	6	6
Sauerkraut	1 c	40	2	0	9	NA	1554	329	2	5	5	3	55	9	7
Spinach	1 c	50	6	1	7	NA	910	513	328	3	15	3	48	24	29
Sweet potato	1 pc	45	1	0	10	NA	19	80	62	1	1	1	10	1	2
Sweet potato, mashed	1 c	275	5	1	63	NA	122	510	398	9	6	8	60	6	11
Tomato	1 c	50	2	0	10	NA	391	523	43	8	4	9	68	1	7

Vegetables, Canned, cont'd.

Food	Serving	Calories	Protein g	Fat g	Carbo g	Fiber g	Sodium mg	Potassium mg	Vit A %rda	Vit B1 %rda (thiamin)	Vit B2 %rda (riboflavin)	Vit B3 %rda (niacin)	Vit C %rda	Calcium %rda	Iron %rda
Tomatoes, baby, sliced, Contadina	1 c	100	2	0	20	NA	660	30	4	4	8	40	16	4	NA
Tomatoes, stewed Hunt	1 c	60	2	0	16	NA	920	20	4	4	8	30	4	4	NA
Tomato puree Contadina	½ c	50	2	0	11	NA	40	25	4	2	6	25	*	4	NA
Water chesnuts La Choy	1 c	65	2	0	15	NA	7	NA	NA	NA	NA	NA	NA	NA	NA

Vegetables, Dry Mixes

Food	Serving	Calories	Protein g	Fat g	Carbo g	Fiber g	Sodium mg	Potassium mg	Vit A %rda	Vit B1 %rda (thiamin)	Vit B2 %rda (riboflavin)	Vit B3 %rda (niacin)	Vit C %rda	Calcium %rda	Iron %rda
Big Tate	½ c	140	2	7	16	NA	410	4	*	2	4	2	2	*	*
Potato Buds, mashed	½ c	130	3	6	15	NA	355	4	*	2	6	2	2	*	*
Potato, mashed French's	½ c	120	2	6	16	NA	365	4	*	2	4	2	2	*	*
Potatoes au gratin French's	½ c	150	3	4	25	NA	525	2	*	6	2	2	10	*	*

Vegetables, Dry Mixes, cont'd.

Food	Serving	Calories	Protein g	Fat g	Carbo g	Fiber g	Sodium mg	Potassium mg	Vit A % rda	Vit B1 % rda (thiamin)	Vit B2 % rda (riboflavin)	Vit B3 % rda (niacin)	Vit C % rda	Calcium % rda	Iron % rda
Potatoes w/sour cream & chive French's	½ c	170	3	7 ●	24	NA	660 ●	NA	2	2	6	4	10 ●	10 ●	*
Potatoes, cheese scalloped French's	½ c	160	4 ●	6 ●	25 ●	NA	540	NA	2	2	8	4	10 ●	10 ●	*

Vegetables, Fresh, Cooked

Food	Serving	Calories	Protein g	Fat g	Carbo g	Fiber g	Sodium mg	Potassium mg	Vit A % rda	Vit B1 % rda (thiamin)	Vit B2 % rda (riboflavin)	Vit B3 % rda (niacin)	Vit C % rda	Calcium % rda	Iron % rda
Artichoke, medium	1	30	3	0 ●	12	NA	36 ●	361 ●	4	5	3	—	17	6	7
Asparagus, cooked	1 c	30	3	0 ●	5	2	2 ●	265 ●	26 ●	15 ●	10 ●	—	63 ●	3	5
Beans, green	1 c	30	2	0 ●	7	4 ●	5 ●	189	14	6	6	—	25 ●	6	4
Beans, wax	1 c	30	2	0 ●	6	NA	4 ●	189	6	6	6	—	27 ●	6	4
Beets, sliced	1 c	55	2	0 ●	12 ●	4 ●	73 ●	354 ●	1	3	4	—	17	2	5
Bok choy	1 c	25	2	0 ●	4	NA	NA	364 ●	105 ●	5	8	—	43 ●	25 ●	6

Vegetables, Fresh, Cooked, cont'd.

Food	Serving	Calories	Protein g	Fat g	Carbo g	Fiber g	Sodium mg	Potassium mg	Vit A %rda	Vit B1 %rda (thiamin)	Vit B2 %rda (riboflavin)	Vit B3 %rda (niacin)	Vit C %rda	Calcium %rda	Iron %rda
Broccoli	1 c	40	5 ●	0 ○	7 ○	6 ●	16 ●	414 ●	78 ●	9 ○	18 ●	6 ●	233 ●	14 ●	7 ○
Brussels sprouts	1 c	55	7 ●	1 ●	10 ○	4 ●	16 ●	423 ●	16 ○	8 ○	13 ●	6 ○	225 ●	5 ○	9 ●
Cabbage, green	1 c	30	2 ○	0 ●	6 ○	4 ●	16 ●	236 ●	4 ○	4 ○	4 ○	2 ○	80 ●	6 ○	2 ○
Carrots	1 c	50	1 ○	0 ○	11 ●	5 ●	51 ●	344 ●	326 ●	5 ○	5 ○	4 ○	15 ○	5 ○	5 ○
Cauliflower	1 c	30	3 ○	0 ●	5 ○	2 ○	13 ●	258 ●	2 ○	7 ○	6 ○	4 ○	115 ●	3 ○	5 ○
Corn on cob, yellow	1	70	2 ○	1 ●	NA	NA	1 ●	151 ○	6 ○	6 ○	5 ○	6 ○	12 ○	0 ○	3 ○
Eggplant, boiled	1 c	38	2 ○	0 ●	8 ○	5 ●	2 ●	300 ●	0 ○	7 ○	5 ○	5 ○	10 ○	2 ○	7 ○
French fries	3 oz	230	3 ○	12 ○	31	NA	NA	726 ●	*	9 ○	3 ○	14 ●	31 ●	2 ○	7 ●
Greens, beet	1 c	25	2 ○	0 ●	5	NA	110 ●	481 ●	148 ●	7 ○	13 ●	2 ○	37 ●	14 ●	16 ●
Greens, collard	1 c	65	7 ●	1 ●	10	NA	24 ●	498 ●	296 ●	14 ●	22 ●	12 ●	240 ●	36 ●	8 ○
Greens, dandelion	1 c	35	2 ○	1 ○	7	NA	46 ●	244 ●	246 ●	9 ○	10 ○	NA	32 ●	15 ●	11 ●

Vegetables, Fresh, Cooked, cont'd.

Food	Serving	Calories	Protein g	Fat g	Carbo g	Fiber g	Sodium mg	Potassium mg	Vit A % rda	Vit B1 % rda (thiamin)	Vit B2 % rda (riboflavin)	Vit B3 % rda (niacin)	Vit C % rda	Calcium % rda	Iron % rda
Greens, mustard	1 c	30	3	1	6	NA	25	308	162	7	12	4	112	19	14
Greens, turnip	1 c	30	3	0	5	NA	NA	NA	165	10	19	4	113	25	8
Kale	1 c	45	5	1	7	5	47	243	183	7	12	4	170	21	10
Okra pods	10	30	2	0	6	3	2	184	10	9	11	9	35	10	3
Onions	1 c	60	3	0	14	4	17	231	*	4	4	2	25	5	4
Parsnips	1 c	100	2	1	23	6	19	587	1	7	7	1	27	7	5
Potato, baked	1	145	4	0	33	4	5	782	*	10	4	14	52	1	6
Potato, boiled	1	105	3	0	23	3	4	556	*	8	3	10	37	1	4
Potato, mashed w/milk	1 c	135	4	2	27	NA	632	548	1	11	6	11	35	44	44
Spinach	1 c	40	5	1	11	6	94	583	292	9	15	5	83	17	22
Squash, summer	1 c	30	2	0	6	5	5	296	16	7	10	9	35	5	4

Vegetables, Fresh, Cooked, cont'd.

Food	Serving	Calories	Protein g	Fat g	Carbo g	Fiber g	Sodium mg	Potassium mg	Vit A %rda	Vit B1 %rda (thiamin)	Vit B2 %rda (riboflavin)	Vit B3 %rda (niacin)	Vit C %rda	Calcium %rda	Iron %rda
Squash, winter	1 c	130	4	1	32	6	2	945	172	7	16	7	45	6	9
Sweet potato, boiled	1	170	3	1	40	4	22	367	239	9	5	5	43	5	6
Sweet potato, baked	1	160	2	1	37	3	17	342	185	7	5	5	42	5	6
Turnips	1 c	35	1	0	8	3	17	291	*	4	5	5	57	5	3
Zucchini, sliced	1 c	22	2	0	5	NA	2	254	11	6	8	7	27	5	4

Vegetables, Frozen, Cooked

Food	Serving	Calories	Protein g	Fat g	Carbo g	Fiber g	Sodium mg	Potassium mg	Vit A %rda	Vit B1 %rda (thiamin)	Vit B2 %rda (riboflavin)	Vit B3 %rda (niacin)	Vit C %rda	Calcium %rda	Iron %rda
Asparagus mornay in pastry Pepperidge Farm	1 pc	250	5	17	18	NA	NA	NA	NA	NA	NA	NA	NA	NA	NA
Asparagus w/butter sauce, Green Giant	1 c	90	3	6	7	NA	1450	25	6	6	15	9	50	2	2
Asparagus, cuts	1 c	40	6	0	6	3	12	396	31	17	14	9	68	4	12

Vegetables, Frozen, Cooked, cont'd.

Food	Serving	Calories	Protein g	Fat g	Carbo g	Fiber g	Sodium mg	Potassium mg	Vit A %rda	Vit B1 %rda (thiamin)	Vit B2 %rda (riboflavin)	Vit B3 %rda (niacin)	Vit C %rda	Calcium %rda	Iron %rda
Bavarian style Birds Eye	1 c	91	4	2	16	NA	518	145	15	4	7	*	15	7	7
Beans, green	1 c	35	2	0	8	4	4	205	16	6	7	3	12	5	5
Beans, green w/almonds Birds Eye	1 c	100	6	4	16	NA	670	330	16	4	8	4	30	8	4
Beans, green w/mushrooms Birds Eye	1 c	52	2	0	12	NA	328	233	14	3	7	*	17	3	3
Beans, green & onion w/bacon bits Green Giant	1 c	80	2	4	9	NA	NA	NA	8	2	6	2	10	2	4
Beans, lima w/butter sauce Green Giant	1 c	220	10	6	32	NA	NA	NA	8	4	2	*	40	6	8
Beans, wax	1 c	35	2	0	8	NA	1	221	3	6	6	3	13	5	5
Broccoli	1 c	50	5	1	9	7	34	392	96	7	13	5	175	10	7
Broccoli w/butter sauce, Green Giant	1 c	90	3	5	8	NA	650	NA	30	4	8	2	100	6	4

Vegetables, Frozen, Cooked, cont'd.

Food	Serving	Calories	Protein g	Fat g	Carbo g	Fiber g	Sodium mg	Potassium mg	Vit A %rda	Vit B1 %rda (thiamin)	Vit B2 %rda (riboflavin)	Vit B3 %rda (niacin)	Vit C %rda	Calcium %rda	Iron %rda
Broccoli w/cheese in pastry Pepperidge Farm	1 pc	250	5	17	19	NA	NA	NA	NA	NA	NA	NA	NA	NA	NA
Broccoli w/cheese sauce, Birds Eye	1 c	340	8	24	24	NA	1330	100	8	20	20	*	120	20	4
Broccoli, carrots & pasta, Birds Eye	1 c	135	3	6	17	NA	390	225	3	3	3	*	68	3	3
Brussels sprouts	1 c	50	5	0	10	4	15	18	8	8	9	5	210	3	7
Brussels sprouts w/butter sauce Green Giant	1 c	110	6	5	10	NA	550	15	6	6	10	2	100	4	4
Brussels sprouts w/cheese sauce Birds Eye	1 c	300	10	20	26	NA	1080	80	12	12	20	4	160	20	8
Carrot nuggets w/butter sauce Green Giant	1 c	100	1	5	12	NA	NA	100	2	2	2	2	15	4	2
Cauliflower	1 c	30	3	0	6	3	18	373	5	5	5	4	123	3	5

Vegetables, Frozen, Cooked, cont'd.

Food	Serving	Calories	Protein g	Fat g	Carbo g	Fiber g	Sodium mg	Potassium mg	Vit A %rda	Vit B1 %rda (thiamin)	Vit B2 %rda (riboflavin)	Vit B3 %rda (niacin)	Vit C %rda	Calcium %rda	Iron %rda
Cauliflower w/cheese sauce Green Giant	1 c	130	6	6	13	NA	NA	40	4	4	2	20	30	4	4
Chinese stir-fry Birds Eye	1 c	68	5	0	16	NA	1136	80	9	9	5	68	14	14	14
Chinese style Birds Eye	1 c	50	4	0	10	NA	630	50	4	4	*	40	4	8	8
Chinese, La Choy	1 c	48	4	1	7	NA	1035	NA	NA	NA	NA	NA	NA	NA	NA
Corn on cob, yellow	1	120	4	1	27	NA	1	9	12	5	11	15	0	6	6
Corn, Niblets w/butter sauce	1 c	190	4	6	30	NA	560	10	4	4	6	15	*	4	4
Corn, green beans & pasta, Birds Eye	1 c	200	6	9	27	NA	509	11	4	4	4	27	11	4	4
Corn, white w/butter sauce Green Giant	1 c	190	4	6	30	NA	NA	*	4	4	10	15	*	2	2
Corn, yellow	1 c	130	5	1	31	9	6	12	10	6	13	13	1	7	7
Cottage fries Birds Eye	3 oz	129	2	5	18	NA	16	*	2	*	6	6	*	2	2

Vegetables, Frozen, Cooked, cont'd.

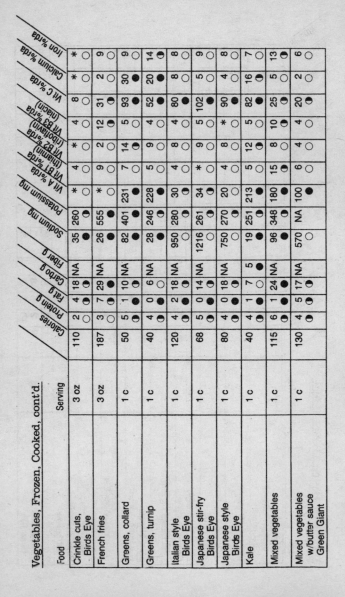

Food	Serving	Calories	Protein g	Fat g	Carbo g	Fiber g	Sodium mg	Potassium mg	Vit A %rda	Vit B1 %rda (thiamin)	Vit B2 %rda (riboflavin)	Vit B3 %rda (niacin)	Vit C %rda	Calcium %rda	Iron %rda
Crinkle cuts, Birds Eye	3 oz	110	2	4	18	NA	35	260	*	4	*	4	8	*	*
French fries	3 oz	187	3	7	29	NA	26	555	*	2	12	31	2	9	9
Greens, collard	1 c	50	5	1	10	NA	82	401	231	14	5	93	30	9	9
Greens, turnip	1 c	40	4	0	6	NA	28	246	228	9	4	52	20	20	14
Italian style, Birds Eye	1 c	120	4	2	18	NA	950	30	5	4	8	80	80	8	8
Japanese stir-fry, Birds Eye	1 c	68	5	0	14	NA	1216	34	4	*	9	102	5	5	9
Japanese style, Birds Eye	1 c	80	4	0	18	NA	750	20	4	4	8	90	4	4	8
Kale	1 c	40	4	1	7	5	19	251	213	5	12	82	16	16	7
Mixed vegetables	1 c	115	6	1	24	NA	96	348	15	10	8	25	5	5	13
Mixed vegetables w/butter sauce Green Giant	1 c	130	4	5	17	NA	570	100	6	4	4	20	2	6	6

Vegetables, Frozen, Cooked, cont'd.

Food	Serving	Calories	Protein g	Fat g	Carbo g	Fiber g	Sodium mg	Potassium mg	Vit A %rda	Vit B1 %rda (thiamin)	Vit B2 %rda (riboflavin)	Vit B3 %rda (niacin)	Vit C %rda	Calcium %rda	Iron %rda
Mixed vegetables w/onion sauce Birds Eye	1 c	262	7	12	31	NA	786	143	10	10	14	24	10	10	*
Mushrooms Dijon in pastry Pepperidge Farm	1 pc	230	3	16	19	NA	NA	NA	NA	NA	NA	NA	NA	NA	NA
Onion Ringers	3 oz	240	3	17	26	NA	188	*	6	3	3	6	3	3	3
Onions w/cheese sauce, Green Giant	1 c	140	3	8	14	NA	800	*	2	*	2	10	8	8	2
Pea pods, Chinese La Choy	6 oz	90	6	0	20	NA	NA	NA	NA	NA	NA	NA	NA	NA	NA
Peas	1 c	110	8	0	19	13	150	19	29	8	8	35	3	3	17
Peas & pea pods w/water chestnuts Le Sueur	1 c	180	5	8	20	NA	820	15	10	6	4	30	4	4	8
Peas & pearl onions Birds Eye	1 c	140	10	0	26	NA	620	30	30	8	16	60	*	8	8
Peas & potatoes w/cream sauce Birds Eye	1 c	420	12	21	45	NA	1440	24	30	24	18	60	12	6	6

Vegetables, Frozen, Cooked, cont'd.

Food	Serving	Calories	Protein g	Fat g	Carbo g	Fiber g	Sodium mg	Potassium mg	Vit A %rda	Vit B1 %rda (thiamin)	Vit B2 %rda (riboflavin)	Vit B3 %rda (niacin)	Vit C %rda	Calcium %rda	Iron %rda
Peas w/cream sauce Birds Eye	1 c	260	8 ○	14 ○	28	NA	880 ○	390 ●	16 ○	20 ●	12 ●	40 ●	8 ○	4 ○	4 ○
Peas, creamed w/bread topping Green Giant	1 c	300	8 ●	15 ○	33 ●	NA	NA	NA	15 ●	10 ●	8 ○	25 ●	20 ●	4 ○	4 ○
Potato, vermicelli Green Giant	1 c	390	11 ●	20 ●	42 ●	NA	NA	NA	6 ○	10 ●	6 ○	10 ○	20 ●	4 ○	4 ○
Potatoes, hash brown	1 c	345	3 ○	18 ●	45 ●	NA	439 ●	439 ○	7 ○	2 ○	8 ●	20 ●	3 ○	11 ●	
Ratatouille, 10 oz, Stouffers	½	60	1 ○	3 ●	9 ○	NA	1317 ○	506 ●	4 ○	4 ○	4 ○	35 ●	2 ○	4 ○	
San Francisco style Birds Eye	1 c	100	4 ●	2 ●	16 ●	NA	610 ●	330 ○	8 ○	8 ●	4 ○	30 ●	30 ●	4 ○	
Spinach	1 c	45	6 ●	1 ●	8 ○	NA	141 ●	683 ●	324 ●	9 ●	4 ○	18 ●	4 ○	65 ●	23 ●	24 ●
Spinach almondine in pastry Pepperidge Farm	1 pc	260	5 ●	18 ○	19 ●	NA	NA	NA	NA	NA	NA	NA	NA	NA	NA
Spinach, creamed Green Giant	1 c	190	6 ●	9 ○	21 ●	NA	NA	50 ●	4 ○	10 ●	2 ○	30 ●	20 ●	10 ●	10 ○
Spinach, w/butter sauce, Green Giant	1 c	90	5 ●	5 ○	6 ○	NA	930 ●	100 ●	2 ○	2 ○	2 ○	60 ●	15 ●	10 ●	10 ●

Vegetables, Frozen, Cooked

Vegetables, Frozen, Cooked, cont'd.

Food	Serving	Calories	Protein g	Fat g	Carbo g	Fiber g	Sodium mg	Potassium mg	Vit A % rda	Vit B1 % rda (thiamin)	Vit B2 % rda (riboflavin)	Vit B3 % rda (niacin)	Vit C % rda	Calcium % rda	Iron % rda
Squash, summer w/cheese sauce Green Giant	1 c	120	4	4	16	NA	NA	15	4	4	4	4	35	4	4
Tasti Puffs	3 oz	143	2	9	14	NA	300	244	3	2	5	4	8	2	2
Tater Tots w/bacon flavor	3 oz	150	3	7	21	NA	610	210	25	*	*	6	8	2	4
Tater Tots w/onions	3 oz	160	2	7	21	NA	550	210	4	*	*	6	8	2	4
Tiny Taters	3 oz	188	2	11	21	NA	263	234	2	*	*	4	6	2	2
Zucchini provencal in pastry Pepperidge Farm	1 pc	210	3	13	21	NA	NA	NA	NA	NA	NA	NA	NA	NA	NA

Vegetables, Raw

Food	Serving	Calories	Protein g	Fat g	Carbo g	Fiber g	Sodium mg	Potassium mg	Vit A % rda	Vit B1 % rda (thiamin)	Vit B2 % rda (riboflavin)	Vit B3 % rda (niacin)	Vit C % rda	Calcium % rda	Iron % rda
Cabbage, green, shredded	1 c	15	1	0	4	2	8	163	2	2	2	1	55	3	2
Cabbage, red	1 c	20	1	0	5	2	18	188	1	2	2	2	72	3	3

Vegetables, Raw, cont'd.

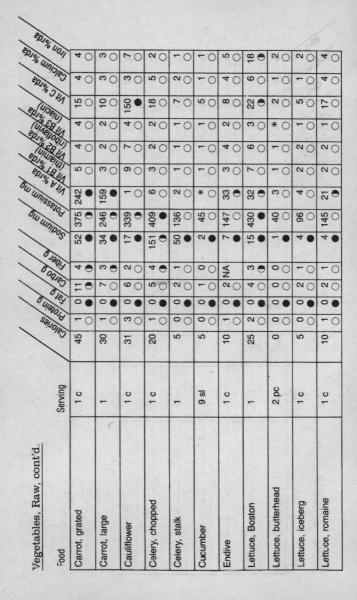

Food	Serving	Calories	Protein g	Fat g	Carbo g	Fiber g	Sodium mg	Potassium mg	Vit A %rda	Vit B1 %rda (thiamin)	Vit B2 %rda (riboflavin)	Vit B3 %rda (niacin)	Vit C %rda	Calcium %rda	Iron %rda
Carrot, grated	1 c	45	1 ○	0 ●	11 ●	4 ●	52 ●	375 ●	242 ●	5 ○	4 ○	4 ○	15 ○	4 ○	4 ○
Carrot, large	1	30	1 ○	0 ●	7 ○	3 ●	34 ●	246 ●	159 ●	3 ○	2 ○	2 ○	10 ○	3 ○	3 ○
Cauliflower	1 c	31	3 ○	0 ●	6 ○	2 ○	17 ○	339 ●	1 ○	9 ○	7 ○	4 ○	150 ●	3 ○	7 ○
Celery, chopped	1 c	20	1 ○	0 ●	5 ○	4 ●	151 ●	409 ●	6 ○	3 ○	2 ○	2 ○	18 ○	5 ○	2 ○
Celery, stalk	1	5	0 ○	0 ●	2 ○	1 ○	50 ●	136 ●	2 ○	1 ○	1 ○	1 ○	7 ○	2 ○	1 ○
Cucumber	9 sl	5	0 ○	0 ●	1 ○	0 ○	2 ●	45 ○	* ○	1 ○	1 ○	1 ○	5 ○	1 ○	1 ○
Endive	1 c	10	1 ○	0 ●	2 ○	NA	7 ●	147 ○	33 ●	3 ○	4 ○	2 ○	8 ○	4 ○	5 ○
Lettuce, Boston	1	25	2 ○	0 ●	4 ○	3 ●	15 ○	430 ●	32 ●	7 ○	6 ○	3 ○	22 ●	6 ○	18 ●
Lettuce, butterhead	2 pc	0	0 ○	0 ●	0 ○	0 ○	1 ●	40 ○	3 ○	1 ○	1 ○	* ○	2 ○	1 ○	2 ○
Lettuce, iceberg	1 c	5	0 ○	0 ●	2 ○	1 ○	4 ●	96 ○	4 ○	2 ○	2 ○	1 ○	5 ○	1 ○	2 ○
Lettuce, romaine	1 c	10	1 ○	0 ●	2 ○	1 ○	4 ●	145 ○	21 ○	2 ○	2 ○	1 ○	17 ○	4 ○	4 ○

Vegetables, Raw, cont'd.

Food	Serving	Calories	Protein g	Fat g	Carbo g	Fiber g	Sodium mg	Potassium mg	Vit A %rda	Vit B1 %rda (thiamin)	Vit B2 %rda (riboflavin)	Vit B3 %rda (niacin)	Vit C %rda	Calcium %rda	Iron %rda
Mushrooms, sliced	1 c	20	2	0	3	2	7	290	*	5	19	15	3	0	3
Onions, chopped	1 c	65	3	0	15	4	17	267	*	3	4	2	28	5	5
Onions, green	6	15	0	0	3	NA	2	69	*	1	1	1	13	1	1
Parsley, chopped	1 tb	0	0	0	0	NA	2	25	6	*	1	*	10	1	1
Radish	4	5	0	0	1	0	2	58	*	1	1	1	8	1	1
Spinach	1 c	15	2	0	2	2	49	259	89	4	6	2	47	5	9
Tomato, medium	1	25	1	0	6	2	15	300	22	5	3	5	47	2	3

Grain Products

Breads

Food	Serving	Calories	Protein g	Fat g	Carbo g	Fiber g	Sodium mg	Potassium mg	Vit A %rda	Vit B1 %rda (thiamin)	Vit B2 %rda (riboflavin)	Vit B3 %rda (niacin)	Vit C %rda	Calcium %rda	Iron %rda
Apple cinnamon Pepperidge Farm	2 sl	140	4	3	26	NA	210	NA	NA	NA	NA	NA	NA	NA	NA
Bran w/raisins Pepperidge Farm	2 sl	130	4	1	25	NA	190	NA	NA	NA	NA	NA	NA	NA	NA
Bran'nola	2 sl	180	7	3	31	NA	355	NA	NA	NA	NA	NA	NA	NA	NA
Cinnamon Pepperidge Farm	2 sl	160	3	4	25	NA	195	NA	NA	NA	NA	NA	NA	NA	NA
Corn & molasses Pepperidge Farm	2 sl	150	3	2	30	NA	260	NA	NA	NA	NA	NA	NA	NA	NA
Cornbread mix Aunt Jemima	1/16	220	5	7	34	NA	600	60	2	*	15	10	10	*	2	8
Cracked wheat Pepperidge Farm	2 sl	150	4	3	26	NA	260	NA	NA	NA	NA	NA	NA	NA	NA
Crumbs, dry	1 c	390	13	5	73	NA	736	152	*	23	21	24	*	12	20	20
Date walnut Pepperidge Farm	2 sl	150	4	5	23	NA	215	NA	NA	NA	NA	NA	NA	NA	NA
French	2 sl	200	6	2	38	2	353	64	*	19	9	12	*	3	9	9
Hollywood dark	2 sl	140	6	2	25	NA	375	NA	0	15	15	10	0	10	15	15

Breads, cont'd.

Food	Serving	Calories	Protein g	Fat g	Carbo g	Fiber g	Sodium mg	Potassium mg	Vit A %rda	Vit B1 %rda (thiamin)	Vit B2 %rda (riboflavin)	Vit B3 %rda (niacin)	Vit C %rda	Calcium %rda	Iron %rda
Hollywood white	2 sl	140	6	2	26	NA	335	NA	0	15	10	10	0	8	10
Italian	2 sl	170	6	0	34	NA	59	44	0	16	8	10	0	1	8
Oatmeal Pepperidge Farm	2 sl	140	4	3	25	NA	370	NA	NA	NA	NA	NA	NA	NA	NA
Profile dark	2 sl	150	6	3	25	NA	310	NA	0	15	8	10	4	4	10
Profile light	2 sl	150	5	2	26	NA	340	NA	0	15	8	10	4	4	10
Pumpernickel, family Pepperidge Farm	2 sl	170	6	2	31	4	610	NA	NA	NA	NA	NA	NA	NA	NA
Pumpernickel, party Pepperidge Farm	4 sl	70	2	1	12	1	220	NA	NA	NA	NA	NA	NA	NA	NA
Raisin	2 sl	130	4	2	26	NA	91	116	*	12	7	6	4	7	NA
Raisin tea Arnold	2 sl	140	3	3	26	NA	225	*	*	6	2	15	4	*	2
Roman Meal	2 sl	140	6	2	27	NA	320	0	0	15	10	10	6	10	10

Breads, cont'd.

Food	Serving	Calories	Protein g	Fat g	Carbo g	Fiber g	Sodium mg	Potassium mg	Vit A % rda	Vit B1 % rda (thiamin)	Vit B2 % rda (riboflavin)	Vit B3 % rda (niacin)	Vit C % rda	Calcium % rda	Iron % rda
Rye, Jewish seeded Arnold	2 sl	150	5 ●	2 ●	28 ●	2 ○	425 ○	NA	* ○	4 ○	2 ○	6 ○	* ○	4 ○	4 ○
Rye, melba thin Arnold	2 sl	100	4 ●	1 ●	19 ●	1 ○	270 ●	NA	* ○	2 ○	2 ○	4 ○	* ○	2 ○	2 ○
Rye, party Pepperidge Farm	4 sl	70	2 ○	1 ●	13 ●	1 ○	415 ●	NA	NA	NA	NA	NA	NA	NA	NA
Rye, seedless Pepperidge Farm	2 sl	170	6 ●	3 ●	31 ●	2 ○	485 ○	NA	NA	NA	NA	NA	NA	NA	NA
Rye, very thin Pepperidge Farm	2 sl	90	2 ○	2 ●	17 ●	1 ○	285 ●	NA	NA	NA	NA	NA	NA	NA	NA
Sprouted wheat Arnold	2 sl	130	5 ●	2 ●	24	NA	265 ●	NA	* ○	10 ●	6 ○	8 ●	* ○	8 ○	8 ○
Vienna Pepperidge Farm	2 sl	150	5 ●	2 ●	27	NA	350 ○	NA	NA	NA	NA	NA	NA	NA	NA
Wheat Fresh Horizons	2 sl	100	5 ●	1 ●	19	6 ●	305 ●	NA	0 ○	15 ●	8 ●	10 ●	0 ○	10 ●	10 ●
Wheat berry Arnold	2 sl	180	6 ●	2 ●	32	NA	410 ○	NA	* ○	15 ●	4 ○	8 ●	* ○	2 ○	10 ●
Wheat germ Pepperidge Farm	2 sl	140	5 ●	2 ●	25	NA	290 ●	NA	NA	NA	NA	NA	NA	10 ●	10 ●
Wheat, butter top Home Pride	2 sl	150	5 ●	3 ●	26	NA	325 ●	NA	0 ○	15 ●	8 ●	10 ●	0 ○	8 ○	8 ○

Breads, cont'd.

Food	Serving	Calories	Protein g	Fat g	Carbo g	Fiber g	Sodium mg	Potassium mg	Vit A %rda	Vit B1 %rda (thiamin)	Vit B2 %rda (riboflavin)	Vit B3 %rda (niacin)	Vit C %rda	Calcium %rda	Iron %rda
White Brick Oven	2 sl	130	4	2	22	1	205	NA	*	8	6	8	*	4	6
White Fresh Horizons	2 sl	100	5	1	19	NA	315	NA	0	15	10	10	0	6	10
White w/buttermilk Wonder	2 sl	150	5	2	27	2	385	NA	0	15	8	10	0	6	8
White, butter top Home Pride	2 sl	150	5	3	26	2	305	NA	0	15	3	10	0	6	8
White, low-sodium Wonder	2 sl	140	4	2	27	2	6	NA	0	15	8	10	0	6	8
White, very thin Pepperidge Farm	2 sl	90	2	2	17	1	175	NA	NA	NA	NA	NA	NA	NA	NA
Whole wheat Brick Oven	2 sl	120	4	3	19	2	190	NA	*	4	4	8	2	6	6
Whole wheat Pepperidge Farm	2 sl	90	3	2	15	2	160	NA	NA	NA	NA	NA	NA	NA	NA
Whole wheat, thin sliced Pepperidge Farm	2 sl	140	4	3	24	3	290	NA	NA	NA	NA	NA	NA	NA	NA

Cereals, Cold

Food	Serving	Calories	Protein g	Fat g	Carbo g	Fiber g	Sodium mg	Potassium mg	Vit A %rda	Vit B1 %rda (thiamin)	Vit B2 %rda (riboflavin)	Vit B3 %rda (niacin)	Vit C %rda	Calcium %rda	Iron %rda
100% Bran Nabisco	⅓ c	47 ○	2 ○	1 ○	14 ○	6 ●	140 ●	NA	*	30 ●	30 ●	30 ●	1 ○	10 ○	10 ○
100% Natural	⅓ c	186 ●	5 ●	8 ○	23 ●	NA	20 ●	153 ○	* ○	5 ○	13 ●	3 ○	3 ○	5 ○	5 ○
100% Natural w/apples & cinnamon	⅓ c	186 ●	4 ●	8 ○	24 ●	4 ●	26 ●	140 ○	* ○	3 ○	5 ○	* ○	5 ○	5 ○	5 ○
100% Natural w/raisins & dates	⅓ c	173 ●	4 ●	7 ●	24 ●	4 ●	20 ●	160 ○	* ○	5 ○	13 ●	* ○	3 ○	5 ○	5 ○
40% bran, Post	⅔ c	90 ○	3 ○	1 ○	23 ●	5 ●	225 ●	165 ○	25 ●	25 ●	25 ●	NA	*	25 ●	25 ●
Alpha-bits	1 c	110 ○	2 ●	1 ●	24 ○	NA	195 ●	55 ○	25 ●	25 ●	25 ●	NA	*	10 ●	10 ○
Apple Jacks	1 c	110 ○	1 ○	0 ●	26 ○	0 ○	115 ●	28 ○	25 ●	25 ●	25 ●	25 ●	0 ○	25 ●	25 ●
Body Buddies, brown sugar & honey	1 c	110 ○	2 ●	1 ●	24 ●	NA	290 ●	NA	25 ●	25 ●	25 ●	25 ●	10 ●	45 ●	45 ●
Body Buddies, fruit flavor	1 c	110 ○	2 ●	1 ●	24 ○	NA	285 ●	NA	25 ●	25 ●	25 ●	25 ●	10 ●	45 ●	45 ●
Boo Berry	1 c	110 ○	1 ●	1 ●	24 ○	NA	210 ●	NA	25 ●	25 ●	25 ●	25 ●	2 ○	25 ●	25 ○
Bran Buds	⅓ c	70 ○	3 ○	1 ●	22 ●	8 ●	185 ●	303 ●	25 ●	25 ●	25 ●	25 ●	2 ○	25 ●	25 ●

Cereals, Cold, cont'd.

Food	Serving	Calories	Protein g	Fat g	Carbo g	Fiber g	Sodium mg	Potassium mg	Vit A %rda	Vit B1 %rda (thiamin)	Vit B2 %rda (riboflavin)	Vit B3 %rda (niacin)	Vit C %rda	Calcium %rda	Iron %rda
Bran Chex	⅔ c	90	3 ○	0 ●	23	6 ●	300 ●	220 ○	* ○	25 ●	25 ●	25 ○	25 ○	* ○	25 ●
Buc Wheats	⅔ c	97	2 ○	1 ●	21	NA	208 ●	NA	40 ●	40 ●	40 ●	40 ●	40 ○	5 ○	40 ●
Cap'n Crunch	1 c	146	1 ○	3 ●	32	NA	223 ●	40 ○	* ○	40 ●	40 ●	40 ●	* ○	* ○	33 ●
Cap'n Crunch w/peanut butter	1 c	173	3 ○	5 ●	28	NA	333 ○	40 ○	* ○	33 ●	33 ●	* ○	* ○	* ○	33 ●
Cheerios	1 c	88	3 ○	2 ●	16	NA	264 ●	NA	20 ●	20 ●	20 ●	20 ●	20 ○	3 ○	20 ●
Cheerios, honey nut	1 c	146	4 ●	1 ●	31	NA	340 ○	NA	33 ●	33 ●	33 ●	33 ●	33 ○	3 ○	33 ●
Chocolate Donutz	1 c	120	2 ○	2 ●	23 ●	NA	185 ●	NA	25 ●	25 ●	25 ●	25 ●	25 ○	* ○	25 ●
Cocoa Pebbles	1 c	126	1 ○	2 ●	29 ●	NA	189 ●	46 ○	* ○	29 ●	29 ●	NA	NA	* ○	11 ○
Cocoa Puffs	1 c	110	1 ○	1 ●	25 ○	NA	205 ●	NA	* ○	25 ●	25 ●	25 ●	25 ○	* ○	25 ●
Cookie Crisp	1 c	110	1 ○	1 ●	25 ○	NA	250 ●	NA	25 ●	25 ●	25 ●	25 ●	25 ○	* ○	25 ●
Corn Bran Quaker	⅔ c	110	2 ○	1 ●	23 ●	NA	295 ●	50 ○	* ○	20 ●	15 ●	* ○	* ○	2 ○	25 ●

Cereals, Cold, cont'd.

Food	Serving	Calories	Protein g	Fat g	Carbo g	Fiber g	Sodium mg	Potassium mg	Vit A %rda	Vit B1 %rda (thiamin)	Vit B2 %rda (riboflavin)	Vit B3 %rda (niacin)	Vit C %rda	Calcium % rda	Iron % rda
Corn Chex	1 c	110 ○	2 ○	0 ●	25 ●	4 ●	310 ●	30 ○	* ○	25 ●	2 ○	25 ●	* ○	10 ●	10 ●
Corn Total	⅔ c	73	1 ○	1 ○	16 ●	NA	206 ●	NA	67 ●	67 ●	67 ●	67 ●	3 ○	67 ●	67 ●
Count Chocula	1 c	110	2 ○	1 ●	24 ●	NA	205 ●	NA	25 ●	25 ●	25 ●	25 ●	2 ○	2 ○	25 ●
Cracklin' Bran	⅔ c	147	3 ○	5 ●	27 ●	5 ●	227 ●	217 ●	34 ●	34 ●	34 ●	33 ●	2 ○	13 ●	25 ●
Crazy Cow, chocolate	1 c	110	1 ○	1 ●	25 ○	NA	185 ●	NA	25 ●	25 ●	25 ●	25 ●	* ○	25 ●	25 ●
Crazy Cow, strawberry	1 c	110	1 ○	1 ●	25 ○	NA	190 ●	NA	25 ●	25 ●	25 ●	25 ●	* ○	25 ●	25 ●
Crispy Wheats 'n Raisins	⅔ c	97	2 ○	1 ●	20 ○	NA	164 ●	NA	22 ●	22 ●	22 ●	* ○	4 ○	22 ●	22 ●
Franken Berry	1 c	110	1 ○	1 ●	24 ○	NA	205 ●	NA	25 ●	25 ●	25 ●	25 ●	2 ○	2 ○	25 ●
Frosted Mini-Wheats	4	110	3 ○	0 ●	24 ●	2 ●	5 ●	73 ○	25 ●	25 ●	25 ●	25 ●	* ○	1 ○	10 ●
Fruit & Fibre, apple cinnamon	⅔ c	120	4 ●	1 ●	29 ●	4 ●	260 ●	207 ●	33 ●	33 ●	33 ●	NA	* ○	33 ●	33 ●
Fruit & Fibre, date raisin	⅔ c	120	4 ●	1 ●	28 ●	4 ●	227 ●	200 ●	33 ●	33 ●	33 ●	NA	* ○	33 ●	33 ●

Cereals, Cold, cont'd.

Food	Serving	Calories	Protein g	Fat g	Carbo g	Fiber g	Sodium mg	Potassium mg	Vit A %rda	Vit B1 %rda (thiamin)	Vit B2 %rda (riboflavin)	Vit B3 %rda (niacin)	Vit C %rda	Calcium %rda	Iron %rda
Fruit Brute	1 c	110	2	1	24	NA	215	NA	25	25	25	25	4	25	25
Golden Grahams	⅔ c	97	2	1	21	NA	306	NA	22	22	22	22	*	22	22
Granola, Post	⅓ c	173	3	5	27	4	73	60	33	33	33	NA	*	33	33
Grape-nuts	⅓ c	133	4	1	31	5	260	113	33	33	33	NA	*	5	5
Grape-nuts flakes	⅔ c	76	2	1	18	3	149	69	19	19	19	NA	*	19	19
Honey Bran	⅔ c	76	2	1	18	NA	152	NA	19	19	19	19	*	19	19
Kaboom	1 c	110	2	1	23	NA	370	NA	45	45	45	45	4	45	45
King Vitaman	1 c	88	2	1	18	NA	240	28	24	32	32	32	*	36	36
Kix	1 c	110	2	1	24	NA	315	NA	25	25	25	25	4	45	45
Life	⅔ c	110	5	1	20	NA	175	100	*	25	25	*	6	25	25
Lucky Charms	1 c	110	2	1	24	NA	185	NA	25	25	25	25	2	25	25

Cereals, Cold, cont'd.

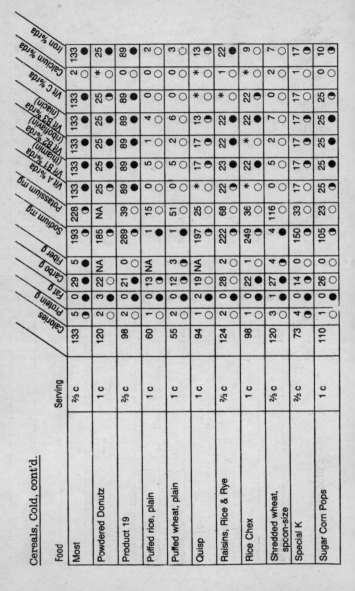

Food	Serving	Calories	Protein g	Fat g	Carbo g	Fiber g	Sodium mg	Potassium mg	Vit A %rda	Vit B1 %rda (thiamin)	Vit B2 %rda (riboflavin)	Vit B3 %rda (niacin)	Vit C %rda	Calcium %rda	Iron %rda
Most	⅔ c	133 ●	5 ●	0 ○	29 ○	5 ●	193 ●	228 ●	133 ●	133 ●	133 ●	133 ●	2 ○	2 ○	133 ●
Powdered Donutz	1 c	120 ○	2 ○	3 ●	22 ●	NA	185 ●	NA	25 ●	25 ●	25 ●	25 ●	* ○	25 ●	25 ●
Product 19	⅔ c	98 ○	2 ○	0 ●	21 ●	0 ○	289 ●	39 ○	89 ●	89 ●	89 ●	89 ●	89 ●	0 ○	89 ●
Puffed rice, plain	1 c	60 ○	1 ○	0 ●	13 ●	NA	1 ●	15 ○	0 ○	5 ○	1 ○	0 ○	0 ○	0 ○	2 ○
Puffed wheat, plain	1 c	55 ○	2 ○	0 ●	12 ●	3 ●	1 ●	51 ○	0 ○	5 ○	2 ○	6 ○	0 ○	3 ○	3 ○
Quisp	1 c	94 ○	1 ○	2 ●	19 ●	NA	197 ●	25 ○	* ○	17 ●	17 ●	13 ●	* ○	13 ●	13 ●
Raisins, Rice & Rye	⅔ c	124 ○	2 ○	0 ●	28 ○	2 ○	222 ●	68 ○	22 ●	23 ●	22 ●	22 ●	1 ○	22 ●	22 ●
Rice Chex	1 c	98 ○	1 ○	0 ●	22 ●	1 ○	249 ●	36 ○	* ○	22 ●	22 ●	22 ●	22 ●	* ○	9 ○
Shredded wheat, spoon-size	⅔ c	120 ○	3 ○	1 ●	27 ●	4 ●	4 ●	116 ○	0 ○	5 ○	2 ○	0 ○	0 ○	2 ○	7 ○
Special K	⅔ c	73 ○	4 ●	0 ●	14 ●	0 ○	150 ●	33 ○	17 ●	17 ●	17 ●	17 ●	2 ○	1 ○	17 ●
Sugar Corn Pops	1 c	110 ○	1 ○	0 ●	26 ○	0 ○	105 ●	23 ○	25 ●	25 ●	25 ●	25 ●	0 ○	0 ○	10 ●

Cereals, Cold, cont'd.

Food	Serving	Calories	Protein g	Fat g	Carbo g	Fiber g	Sodium mg	Potassium mg	Vit A % rda	Vit B1 % rda (thiamin)	Vit B2 % rda (riboflavin)	Vit B3 % rda (niacin)	Vit C % rda	Calcium % rda	Iron % rda
Super Sugar Crisp	1 c	126	2	1	30	NA	40	51	29	29	29	29	NA	*	11
Team	2/3 c	73	1	1	16	NA	123	NA	17	17	17	17	17	*	5
Total	2/3 c	73	2	1	15	2	250	NA	67	67	67	67	67	3	67
Trix	1 c	110	1	1	25	NA	170	NA	25	25	25	25	25	*	25
Wheat Chex	2/3 c	110	3	0	23	3	200	115	*	25	4	25	*	*	25
Wheat flakes w/sugar	1 c	105	3	0	24	4	380	81	26	27	26	27	27	1	27
Wheat germ, plain	1 tb	25	2	1	3	1	0	57	0	7	3	2	2	0	3
Wheaties	2/3 c	73	2	1	15	2	246	NA	17	17	17	17	17	3	17

Cereals, Hot, Prepared

Food	Serving	Calories	Protein g	Fat g	Carbo g	Fiber g	Sodium mg	Potassium mg	Vit A %rda	Vit B1 %rda (thiamin)	Vit B2 %rda (riboflavin)	Vit B3 %rda (niacin)	Vit C %rda	Calcium %rda	Iron %rda
Cream of wheat, apple cinnamon Mix 'n Eat	1 pk	130	3 ○	0 ●	29 ●	NA	240 ●	NA	25 ●	25 ●	15 ●	25 ●	* ○	2 ○	45 ●
Cream of wheat, quick	⅔ c	76	2 ○	0 ●	16 ●	NA	130 ●	* ○	8 ○	8 ○	3 ○	5 ○	* ○	11 ●	34 ●
Cream of wheat, reg	⅔ c	76	2 ○	0 ●	17 ●	NA	10 ●	* ○	8 ○	8 ○	3 ○	5 ○	* ○	* ○	34 ●
Cream of wheat, reg Mix 'n Eat	1 pk	100	3 ○	0 ●	21 ●	NA	240 ●	25 ●	NA	25 ●	15 ●	25 ●	* ○	2 ○	45 ●
Cream of wheat, instant	⅔ c	100	3 ○	0 ●	21 ●	NA	10 ●	* ○	10 ●	10 ●	4 ○	6 ○	* ○	15 ●	45 ●
Farina	1 c	105	3 ○	0 ●	22 ●	1 ○	1 ●	25 ○	0 ○	8 ○	4 ○	5 ○	0 ○	15 ●	28 ●
Grits, corn	1 c	125	3 ○	0 ●	27 ●	4 ●	1 ●	27 ○	0 ○	7 ○	4 ○	5 ○	0 ○	0 ○	4 ○
Grits, instant, plain, Quaker	1 pk	80	2 ○	0 ●	18 ●	NA	520 ○	10 ○	0 ○	8 ○	4 ○	4 ○	* ○	* ○	4 ○
Grits, instant, w/imitation ham Quaker	1 pk	100	3 ○	0 ●	21 ●	NA	895 ○	15 ○	0 ○	8 ○	4 ○	4 ○	* ○	* ○	4 ○
Grits, quick Quaker	3 tb	100	2 ○	0 ●	22 ●	NA	9 ●	10 ○	0 ○	8 ○	4 ○	4 ○	* ○	* ○	4 ○

Cereals, Hot, Prepared, cont'd.

Food	Serving	Calories	Protein g	Fat g	Carbo g	Fiber g	Sodium mg	Potassium mg	Vit A %rda	Vit B1 %rda (thiamin)	Vit B2 %rda (riboflavin)	Vit B3 %rda (niacin)	Vit C %rda	Calcium %rda	Iron %rda
Oatmeal	1 c	130	5	2	23	6	1	146	0	13	3	1	0	2	8
Oats, instant, apple cinnamon Quaker	1 pk	140	4	2	26	NA	260	60	20	20	10	15	*	10	25
Oats, instant, bran raisin Quaker	1 pk	150	4	2	29	NA	340	120	20	20	10	15	*	10	25
Oats, instant, raisin spice Quaker	1 pk	160	4	2	31	NA	310	80	20	20	10	15	*	10	25
Oats, instant, regular, Quaker	1 pk	110	4	2	18	NA	400	50	20	20	10	15	*	10	25
Oats, old-fashioned Quaker	⅔ c	110	5	2	18	NA	9	55	10	10	*	*	*	*	4
Oats, quick Quaker	⅔ c	110	5	2	18	NA	9	55	10	10	*	*	*	*	4
Wheat	1 c	110	4	1	23	NA	2	118	10	3	3	8	0	2	7
Whole wheat natural Quaker	⅔ c	100	3	1	21	NA	9	55	6	4	2	4	*	*	4

Crackers (approx. 1 oz)

Food	Serving	Calories	Protein g	Fat g	Carbo g	Fiber g	Sodium mg	Potassium mg	Vit A %rda	Vit B1 %rda (thiamin)	Vit B2 %rda (riboflavin)	Vit B3 %rda (niacin)	Vit C %rda	Calcium %rda	Iron %rda
Arrowroot biscuit National	6	130	2	4	21	NA	100	NA	*	6	4	2	*	*	2
Cheese Nips	26	140	3	6	18	NA	360	NA	*	10	8	8	*	2	4
Cheese Tid-bit	32	150	2	9	16	NA	430	NA	8	8	6	6	*	4	4
Chicken in a Biskit	14	150	2	9	16	NA	260	NA	6	6	4	4	*	*	4
Chocolate graham Nabisco	3	170	2	8	21	NA	NA	NA	*	*	4	4	*	*	6
English water biscuit Pepperidge Farm	7	120	3	3	22	NA	170	NA	NA	NA	NA	NA	NA	NA	NA
Escort	7	150	2	8	18	NA	240	NA	8	8	6	6	*	*	4
French onion Nabisco	12	150	2	7	18	NA	280	NA	8	8	6	6	*	4	4
Graham	2	55	1	1	10	1	96	55	0	1	5	3	0	1	3
Melba toast	7 pc	105	4	1	19	NA	21	63	NA	NA	NA	NA	NA	NA	NA

Crackers (approx. 1 oz), cont'd.

Food	Serving	Calories	Protein g	Fat g	Carbo g	Fiber g	Sodium mg	Potassium mg	Vit A %rda	Vit B1 %rda (thiamin)	Vit B2 %rda (riboflavin)	Vit B3 %rda (niacin)	Vit C %rda	Calcium %rda	Iron %rda
Oysterettes	36	120	3	3	20	NA	440	NA	*	6	6	6	*	*	6
Rich & Crisp	10	140	2	6	19	NA	300	NA	*	10	6	6	*	2	4
Ritz	9	150	2	8	18	NA	270	NA	*	6	6	6	*	4	4
RyKrisp, natural	2	50	1	0	10	NA	110	NA	*	2	*	*	*	*	2
RyKrisp, seasoned	2	60	1	1	9	NA	220	NA	*	2	*	*	*	*	2
RyKrisp, sesame	2	60	1	2	10	NA	220	NA	*	2	2	*	*	*	2
Rye	2	45	2	0	10	2	151	78	*	3	0	1	0	1	3
Saltine	10	122	2	2	20	1	312	32	0	8	7	5	0	1	7
Sesame Wheats!	9	150	2	9	16	NA	250	NA	*	8	4	6	*	4	6
Snacks Ahoy	15	140	2	7	17	NA	NA	NA	*	6	4	4	*	*	2
Sociables	14	150	3	7	18	NA	330	NA	*	10	6	6	*	4	6

Crackers (approx. 1 oz.), cont'd.

Food	Serving	Calories	Protein g	Fat g	Carbo g	Fiber g	Sodium mg	Potassium mg	Vit A %rda	Vit B1 %rda (thiamin)	Vit B2 %rda (riboflavin)	Vit B3 %rda (niacin)	Vit C %rda	Calcium %rda	Iron %rda
Swiss cheese Nabisco	15	150	3	8	17	NA	330	NA	*	10	8	6	*	4	4
Triscuit	7	140	3	5	21	NA	180	NA	*	4	2	6	*	*	4
Uneeda biscuits, unsalted top	6	130	3	4	22	NA	230	NA	*	8	8	8	*	*	8
Vegetable Thins	13	150	2	8	17	NA	300	NA	*	8	6	6	*	4	4
Waverly wafers	8	140	2	6	21	NA	310	NA	*	8	6	6	*	4	4
Wheat Thins	16	140	2	6	19	NA	240	NA	*	6	4	6	*	*	4
Wheatsworth	9	130	3	6	16	NA	330	NA	*	10	6	6	*	2	6
Zweiback Nabisco	4	120	3	3	21	NA	80	NA	*	6	8	4	*	*	4

Flour

Food	Serving	Calories	Protein g	Fat g	Carbo g	Fiber g	Sodium mg	Potassium mg	Vit A %rda	Vit B1 %rda (thiamin)	Vit B2 %rda (riboflavin)	Vit B3 %rda (niacin)	Vit C %rda	Calcium %rda	Iron %rda
Better for Bread	1 c	400	14	1	83	NA	4	NA	*	45	25	30	*	2	20
Bisquick	1 c	480	8	16	76	NA	1400	NA	*	30	20	20	*	16	12
Bread, Pillsbury	1 c	410	14	3	81	NA	4	NA	0	50	25	30	0	2	20
Buckwheat	1 c	340	6	1	78	NA	NA	314	0	5	2	2	0	1	6
Cake	1 c	350	7	1	76	2	3	91	0	41	22	26	0	2	16
Cornmeal	1 c	500	11	2	108	NA	1	166	12	41	21	24	0	1	22
Masa harina Quaker	1 c	420	9	3	81	NA	27	90	*	60	30	30	0	12	24
Masa trigo Quaker	1 c	450	9	12	75	NA	885	27	*	45	24	24	*	18	18
Rye and wheat, Bohemian style Pillsbury	1 c	400	11	1	86	NA	4	NA	0	20	10	15	0	2	8
Self-rising Gold Medal	1 c	380	10	1	83	NA	1520	NA	*	45	25	30	*	20	20

Flour, cont'd.

Food	Serving	Calories	Protein g	Fat g	Carbo g	Fiber g	Sodium mg	Potassium mg	Vit A %rda	Vit B1 %rda (thiamin)	Vit B2 %rda (riboflavin)	Vit B3 %rda (niacin)	Vit C %rda	Calcium %rda	Iron %rda
White	1 c	455	13	1	95	4	3	119	0	53	29	33	0	2	20
Whole wheat	1 c	400	16	2	85	11	4	444	0	44	8	26	0	5	22
Wondra	1 c	400	11	1	87	NA	4	NA	*	45	25	30	*	2	20

Grains

Food	Serving	Calories	Protein g	Fat g	Carbo g	Fiber g	Sodium mg	Potassium mg	Vit A %rda	Vit B1 %rda (thiamin)	Vit B2 %rda (riboflavin)	Vit B3 %rda (niacin)	Vit C %rda	Calcium %rda	Iron %rda
Barley, pearled Quaker	1 c	170	5	1	36	NA	9	30	*	4	*	8	*	4	4
Barley, pearled, raw	1 c	700	16	2	158	13	2	320	0	16	6	31	0	3	22
Barley, quick Quaker	1 c	226	7	1	48	NA	12	40	*	5	*	11	*	*	5
Bulghur, canned, seasoned	1 c	245	8	4	44	NA	621	151	0	5	3	21	0	3	11

Muffins

Food	Serving	Calories	Protein g	Fat g	Carbo g	Fiber g	Sodium mg	Potassium mg	Vit A %rda	Vit B1 %rda (thiamin)	Vit B2 %rda (riboflavin)	Vit B3 %rda (niacin)	Vit C %rda	Calcium %rda	Iron %rda
Blueberry	1	110 ○	4 ●	17 ●	NA	NA	253 ○	46 ○	2 ○	6 ○	6 ○	4 ○	* ○	3 ○	3 ○
Bran'nola	1	160 ●	1 ●	30 ●	NA	NA	260 ●	NA	10 ●	10 ●	10 ●	8 ○	* ○	6 ○	10 ●
Cinnamon w/apple Pepperidge Farm	1	140 ●	2 ●	27 ●	NA	NA	350 ○	NA	NA	NA	NA	NA	NA	NA	NA
Cinnamon w/raisins Pepperidge Farm	1	150 ●	2 ●	28 ●	NA	NA	355 ○	NA	NA	NA	NA	NA	NA	NA	NA
Corn	1	125 ○	4 ●	19 ●	NA	NA	192 ●	54 ○	7 ○	6 ○	6 ○	4 ○	* ○	4 ○	4 ○
English, Thomas'	1	130 ●	4 ●	26 ●	NA	NA	215 ●	NA	15 ●	8 ○	8 ○	8 ○	* ○	4 ○	7 ○
Extra crisp Arnold	1	150 ○	1 ●	30 ●	NA	NA	310 ○	NA	25 ●	15 ●	15 ●	10 ●	* ○	2 ○	10 ●
Plain	1	120 ○	4 ●	17 ●	NA	NA	176 ○	50 ○	6 ○	7 ○	5 ○	5 ○	* ○	4 ○	3 ○
Popover mix, Flako	1 pc	170 ●	5 ●	25 ●	NA	NA	355 ●	110 ○	6 ○	8 ○	8 ○	2 ○	* ○	6 ○	4 ○
Raisin Arnold	1	170 ●	1 ●	35 ●	NA	NA	350 ○	NA	20 ●	10 ●	10 ●	10 ●	* ○	6 ○	10 ●

Muffins, cont'd.

Food	Serving	Calories	Protein g	Fat g	Carbo g	Fiber g	Sodium mg	Potassium mg	Vit A %rda	Vit B1 %rda (thiamin)	Vit B2 %rda (riboflavin)	Vit B3 %rda (niacin)	Vit C %rda	Calcium %rda	Iron %rda
Wheat, stone ground Pepperidge Farm	1	130	5	2	25	NA	340	NA	NA	NA	NA	NA	NA	NA	NA
Wild blueberry Duncan Hines	1	110	2	3	17	NA	180	NA	*	*	2	*	*	2	2

Pancakes, Prep (4-inch)

Food	Serving	Calories	Protein g	Fat g	Carbo g	Fiber g	Sodium mg	Potassium mg	Vit A %rda	Vit B1 %rda (thiamin)	Vit B2 %rda (riboflavin)	Vit B3 %rda (niacin)	Vit C %rda	Calcium %rda	Iron %rda
Blueberry batter, frozen, Aunt Jemima	3	210	5	3	44	NA	905	75	*	15	10	6	*	4	4
Buckwheat mix Aunt Jemima	3	200	7	8	25	NA	520	145	4	10	10	6	*	15	6
Buttermilk batter, frozen, Aunt Jemima	3	210	7	2	43	NA	950	105	*	20	15	8	*	8	8
Buttermilk mix Aunt Jemima	3	300	10	11	40	NA	990	155	6	20	20	10	*	30	10
Complete mix Aunt Jemima	3	240	6	3	47	NA	870	60	*	20	10	10	*	10	8
Extra Lights	3	200	6	7	28	NA	495	NA	4	15	15	6	0	15	4
Panshakes	3	250	8	6	40	NA	855	NA	2	20	20	10	0	15	8

Pancakes, Prep (4-inch), cont'd.

Food	Serving	Calories	Protein g	Fat g	Carbo g	Fiber g	Sodium mg	Potassium mg	Vit A %rda	Vit B1 %rda (thiamin)	Vit B2 %rda (riboflavin)	Vit B3 %rda (niacin)	Vit C %rda	Calcium %rda	Iron %rda
Potato, from mix French's	3	130	3	5	17	NA	490	NA	2	*	4	4	10	2	2
Regular batter, frozen, Aunt Jemima	3	210	7	3	43	NA	1110	75	*	20	10	8	4	*	0
Regular mix Aunt Jemima	3	220	7	8	26	NA	550	135	4	10	10	2	15	15	6
Whole wheat mix Aunt Jemima	3	250	10	9	32	NA	725	210	4	10	15	10	20	20	10

Pasta

Food	Serving	Calories	Protein g	Fat g	Carbo g	Fiber g	Sodium mg	Potassium mg	Vit A %rda	Vit B1 %rda (thiamin)	Vit B2 %rda (riboflavin)	Vit B3 %rda (niacin)	Vit C %rda	Calcium %rda	Iron %rda
Macaroni, cooked elbow, twist, shell	1 c	155	5	1	32	2	85	0	0	13	6	8	0	1	7
Noodles, chow mein La Choy	½ c	153	3	9	16	NA	201	NA	NA	NA	NA	NA	NA	NA	NA
Noodles, egg, cooked	1 c	200	7	2	37	2	70	2	2	15	8	10	0	2	8
Rice noodles La Choy	½ c	130	2	5	20	NA	359	NA	NA	NA	NA	NA	NA	NA	NA
Spaghetti, cooked	1 c	155	5	1	32	2	85	1	0	13	6	8	0	1	7

Rice and Rice Dishes

Food	Serving	Calories	Protein g	Fat g	Carbo g	Fiber g	Sodium mg	Potassium mg	Vit A %rda	Vit B1 %rda (thiamin)	Vit B2 %rda (riboflavin)	Vit B3 %rda (niacin)	Vit C %rda	Calcium %rda	Iron %rda
Beef mix, Minute	½ c	150	3 ○	4 ◐	25 ●	NA	720 ○	25 ○	2 ○	20 ●	* ○	8 ○	* ○	* ○	6 ○
Brown & wild w/o butter Uncle Ben's	½ c	126	4 ◐	2 ●	25 ●	NA	474 ○	200 ◐	1 ○	7 ○	4 ○	10 ○	2 ◐	1 ○	6 ○
Brown, Converted w/o butter/salt	½ c	100	3 ○	1 ●	20 ●	NA	4 ●	74 ○	0 ○	7 ○	1 ○	8 ○	0 ○	1 ○	4 ○
Chicken mix, Minute	½ c	150	3 ○	4 ◐	25 ●	NA	685 ○	20 ○	2 ○	15 ◐	* ○	8 ○	* ○	* ○	6 ○
Chinese fried Minute	½ c	160	3 ○	5 ◐	25 ●	NA	635 ○	45 ○	* ○	15 ◐	* ○	8 ○	* ○	* ○	6 ○
Chinese style La Choy	½ c	207	4 ◐	2 ●	43 ●	NA	1225 ○	NA	NA	NA	NA	NA	NA	NA	NA
Continental Green Giant	½ c	115	2 ○	4 ◐	18 ◐	NA	NA	NA	4 ○	8 ○	3 ○	5 ○	4 ○	2 ○	5 ○
Fried, chicken La Choy	½ c	209	7 ◐	2 ●	40 ●	NA	1153 ○	NA	NA	NA	NA	NA	NA	NA	NA
Long grain & wild w/o butter Uncle Ben's	½ c	97	3 ○	0 ●	21 ●	NA	420 ○	93 ○	1 ○	7 ○	2 ○	6 ○	0 ○	3 ○	6 ○

Rice and Rice Dishes, cont'd.

Food	Serving	Calories	Protein g	Fat g	Carbo g	Fiber g	Sodium mg	Potassium mg	Vit A %rda	Vit B1 %rda (thiamin)	Vit B2 %rda (riboflavin)	Vit B3 %rda (niacin)	Vit C %rda	Calcium %rda	Iron %rda
Long grain & wild, quick, w/o butter Uncle Ben's	½ c	95	3	1	20	NA	387	0	7	1	5	2	2	1	6
Pilaf Green Giant	½ c	115	2	2	23	NA	520	*	5	1	5	2	*	*	4
Rice 'n broccoli w/cheese sauce Green Giant	½ c	125	3	4	20	NA	405	23	8	1	8	30	4	4	5
Rice, instant, cooked	½ c	90	2	0	20	1	6	0	7	*	4	0	0	0	4
Rice, long-grain, cooked	½ c	113	2	0	25	1	3	29	8	1	5	0	1	1	5
Rice, long-grain, raw	½ c	335	6	1	75	2	5	85	27	2	16	0	2	15	15
Rice-A-Roni, Spanish	½ c	80	2	1	17	NA	NA	*	10	4	7	*	NA	4	4
Rice-A-Roni, beef	½ c	130	3	1	27	NA	NA	*	25	8	8	*	NA	6	6
Verdi, Green Giant	½ c	135	2	4	24	NA	500	1	8	2	4	2	1	1	5

Rice and Rice Dishes, cont'd.

Food	Serving	Calories	Protein g	Fat g	Carbo g	Fiber g	Sodium mg	Potassium mg	Vit A %rda	Vit B1 %rda (thiamin)	Vit B2 %rda (riboflavin)	Vit B3 %rda (niacin)	Vit C %rda	Calcium %rda	Iron %rda
White & wild Oriental Green Giant	½ c	115	2	3	20	NA	NA	NA	2	10	2	4	13	1	5
White, Converted w/o butter/salt	½ c	97	2	0	22	NA	2	41	0	8	1	6	0	3	5

Rolls and Croissants

Food	Serving	Calories	Protein g	Fat g	Carbo g	Fiber g	Sodium mg	Potassium mg	Vit A %rda	Vit B1 %rda (thiamin)	Vit B2 %rda (riboflavin)	Vit B3 %rda (niacin)	Vit C %rda	Calcium %rda	Iron %rda
Bagel, egg	1	165	6	2	28	NA	NA	41	1	9	6	6	0	1	7
Bagel, water	1	165	6	1	30	NA	NA	42	0	10	6	7	0	1	7
Biscuit, Butter tastin' Hungry Jack	2	190	3	10	22	NA	550	NA	0	10	6	8	0	0	6
Biscuit, Extra Lights	2	120	3	3	21	NA	525	NA	0	8	2	4	0	0	4
Biscuit, Heat 'n Eat	2	200	3	11	23	NA	565	NA	0	15	8	8	0	0	4

Rolls and Croissants, cont'd.

Food	Serving	Calories	Protein g	Fat g	Carbo g	Fiber g	Sodium mg	Potassium mg	Vit A %rda	Vit B1 %rda (thiamin)	Vit B2 %rda (riboflavin)	Vit B3 %rda (niacin)	Vit C %rda	Calcium %rda	Iron %rda
Biscuit, baking powder 1869 Brand	2	200	4	9	27	NA	585	NA	10	10	10	8	0	0	6
Biscuit, buttermilk extra rich Hungry Jack	2	130	2	6	18	NA	410	NA	8	4	4	4	0	0	2
Biscuit, flaky Hungry Jack	2	180	3	9	23	NA	580	NA	10	6	8	8	0	0	4
Brown 'n serve, French Pepperidge Farm	2 oz	180	6	2	34	NA	470	NA	NA	NA	NA	NA	NA	NA	NA
Brown 'n serve, Italian Pepperidge Farm	2 oz	150	4	3	27	NA	320	NA	NA	NA	NA	NA	NA	NA	NA
Butter crescent Pepperidge Farm	1	110	2	6	14	NA	165	NA							
Crescent Pillsbury	2	200	4	10	24	NA	665	NA	10	4	4	4	0	0	4
Dinner party Arnold	2	110	3	3	20	1	280	*	4	4	4	4	*	6	6
Finger w/poppy seed Pepperidge Farm	1	60	1	2	9	NA	120	NA	NA	NA	NA	NA	NA	NA	NA

Rolls and Croissants, cont'd.

Food	Serving	Calories	Protein g	Fat g	Carbo g	Fiber g	Sodium mg	Potassium mg	Vit A %rda	Vit B1 %rda (thiamin)	Vit B2 %rda (riboflavin)	Vit B3 %rda (niacin)	Vit C %rda	Calcium %rda	Iron %rda
French style Pepperidge Farm	1	110	3○	2●	20●	NA	245●	NA	NA	NA	NA	NA	NA	NA	NA
Golden twist Pepperidge Farm	1	120	2○	6●	20●	NA	160●	NA	NA	NA	NA	NA	NA	NA	NA
Hard	1	155	5●	2●	30●	NA	313●	49○	*○	13●	7○	9○	*○	2○	7○
Hotdog/hamburger	1	120	3○	2●	21●	NA	202●	38○	*○	11●	6○	7○	*○	3○	4○
Parker house Pepperidge Farm	1	60	1○	2●	9○	1○	95●	NA	NA	NA	NA	NA	NA	NA	NA
Sandwich, onion w/poppy Pepperidge Farm	1	150	5●	3●	27●	NA	285●	NA	NA	NA	NA	NA	NA	NA	NA
Scurdough French Arnold	1	90	3○	1●	16●	NA	160●	*○	*○	10●	4○	4○	*○	*○	6○
Submarine	1	390	12●	4●	75●	NA	783○	*○	*○	36●	19●	23●	6○	6○	17●

Stuffings and Croutons

Food	Serving	Calories	Protein g	Fat g	Carbo g	Fiber g	Sodium mg	Potassium mg	Vit A %rda	Vit B1 %rda (thiamin)	Vit B2 %rda (riboflavin)	Vit B3 %rda (niacin)	Vit C %rda	Calcium %rda	Iron %rda
Croutons, cheddar & romano Pepperidge Farm	½ oz	60	1	3	10	NA	185	NA	NA	NA	NA	NA	NA	NA	NA
Croutons, cheese & garlic Pepperidge Farm	½ oz	70	1	3	9	NA	175	NA	NA	NA	NA	NA	NA	NA	NA
Croutons, onion & garlic Pepperidge Farm	½ oz	70	1	3	10	NA	160	NA	NA	NA	NA	NA	NA	NA	NA
Croutons, sour cream & chive Pepperidge Farm	½ oz	70	1	3	9	NA	185	NA	NA	NA	NA	NA	NA	NA	NA
Croutons, seasoned Pepperidge Farm	½ oz	70	1	3	9	NA	215	NA	NA	NA	NA	NA	NA	NA	NA
Stuffing, New England Stove-top	½ c	180	4	9	21	NA	630	6	10	6	6	*	*	4	4
Stuffing, chicken Stove-top	½ c	170	4	9	20	NA	635	6	8	4	6	*	4	4	4
Stuffing, cornbread Stove-top	½ c	170	3	8	22	NA	550	6	6	4	4	*	*	4	4

Stuffings and Croutons, cont'd.

Food	Serving	Calories	Protein g	Fat g	Carbo g	Fiber g	Sodium mg	Potassium mg	Vit A % rda	Vit B1 % rda (thiamin)	Vit B2 % rda (riboflavin)	Vit B3 % rda (niacin)	Vit C % rda	Calcium % rda	Iron % rda
Stuffing, cube Pepperidge Farm	½ c	160	3	8	22	NA	580	NA	NA	NA	NA	NA	NA	NA	NA
Stuffing, cube, unseasoned Pepperidge Farm	½ c	160	3	8	22	NA	580	NA	NA	NA	NA	NA	NA	NA	NA
Stuffing, herb Pepperidge Farm	½ c	160	3	8	22	NA	590	NA	NA	NA	NA	NA	NA	NA	NA
Stuffing, pan, seasoned Pepperidge Farm	½ c	160	3	7	23	NA	580	NA	NA	NA	NA	NA	NA	NA	NA
Stuffing, w/rice Stove-top	½ c	180	3	9	23	NA	505	70	6	8	2	6	*	2	4

Waffles

Food	Serving	Calories	Protein g	Fat g	Carbo g	Fiber g	Sodium mg	Potassium mg	Vit A % rda	Vit B1 % rda (thiamin)	Vit B2 % rda (riboflavin)	Vit B3 % rda (niacin)	Vit C % rda	Calcium % rda	Iron % rda
Blueberry, jumbo, frozen, Aunt Jemima	1	80	2	2	14	NA	315	35	*	10	10	10	*	4	10
Buttermilk, jumbo, frozen, Aunt Jemima	1	80	2	2	14	NA	350	30	*	10	10	10	*	4	10
From mix	1	205	7	8	27	1	515	146	3	9	13	5	18	6	6

Waffles, cont'd.

Food	Serving	Calories	Protein g	Fat g	Carbo g	Fiber g	Sodium mg	Potassium mg	Vit A %rda	Vit B1 %rda (thiamin)	Vit B2 %rda (riboflavin)	Vit B3 %rda (niacin)	Vit C %rda	Calcium %rda	Iron %rda
Hot 'n Buttery Downyflake	1	65	2	3	11	NA	NA	NA	*	5	4	4	*	*	5
Original, jumbo, frozen, Aunt Jemima	1	80	2	2	14	NA	340	35	*	10	10	10	*	4	10

Meat, Poultry & Fish
Beef, Fresh

Food	Serving	Calories	Protein g	Fat g	Carbo g	Fiber g	Sodium mg	Potassium mg	Vit A %rda	Vit B1 %rda (thiamin)	Vit B2 %rda (riboflavin)	Vit B3 %rda (niacin)	Vit C %rda	Calcium %rda	Iron % rda
Ground round	4 oz	247 ●	31 ●	13 ○	0 ○	0 ○	76 ●	348 ●	1 ○	7 ○	16 ●	34 ●	NA	1 ○	22 ●
Ground, regular	4 oz	313 ●	27 ●	23 ○	0 ○	0 ○	67 ●	295 ●	1 ○	6 ○	13 ●	29 ●	NA	1 ○	19 ●
Hamburger Helper, beef romanoff, prepared	⅕	340 ●	21 ●	16 ○	28 ●	NA	1095 ○	NA	*○	20 ●	15 ●	25 ●	*○	6 ○	15 ●
Hamburger Helper, chili tomato, prepared	⅕	320 ●	19 ●	14 ○	29 ●	NA	1230 ○	NA	8 ○	20 ●	15 ●	25 ●	*○	2 ○	20 ●
Hamburger Helper, lasagne, prepared	⅕	330 ●	19 ●	14 ○	33 ●	NA	1000 ○	NA	10 ○	20 ●	15 ●	25 ●	*○	2 ○	15 ●
Hamburger Helper, tamale pie, prepared	⅕	370 ●	19 ●	15 ○	39 ●	NA	910 ○	NA	6 ○	20 ●	15 ●	25 ●	*○	4 ○	15 ●
Liver, fried	4 oz	260 ●	29 ●	12 ○	7 ○	0 ○	133 ●	1210 ●	20 ●	20 ●	279 ●	93 ●	51 ●	1 ○	56 ●
Rib roast, untrimmed	4 oz	500 ●	23 ○	44 ○	0 ○	0 ○	55 ●	252 ●	4 ○	10 ●	21 ●	NA	1 ○	16 ●
Rib roast, trimmed	4 oz	278 ●	31 ○	16 ○	0 ○	0 ○	78 ●	358 ●	6 ○	14 ●	29 ●	NA	1 ○	22 ●

Beef, Fresh, cont'd.

Food	Serving	Calories	Protein g	Fat g	Carbo g	Fiber g	Sodium mg	Potassium mg	Vit A % rda	Vit B1 % rda (thiamin)	Vit B2 % rda (riboflavin)	Vit B3 % rda (niacin)	Vit C % rda	Calcium % rda	Iron % rda
Round roast, trimmed	4 oz	179	34	4	0	0	72	383	*	6	15	31	NA	1	24
Round roast, untrimmed	4 oz	220	33	9	0	0	80	372	0	5	15	30	NA	2	24
Round steak, trimmed	4 oz	217	35	7	0	0	87	397	0	6	16	34	NA	2	23
Round steak, untrimmed	4 oz	293	32	17	0	0	80	363	1	6	15	32	NA	1	22
Sirloin steak, trimmed	4 oz	230	36	8	0	0	83	404	0	7	16	36	NA	1	24
Sirloin steak, untrimmed	4 oz	440	27	36	0	0	53	293	1	4	12	27	NA	1	19

Beef, Processed

Food	Serving	Calories	Protein g	Fat g	Carbo g	Fiber g	Sodium mg	Potassium mg	Vit A % rda	Vit B1 % rda (thiamin)	Vit B2 % rda (riboflavin)	Vit B3 % rda (niacin)	Vit C % rda	Calcium % rda	Iron % rda
Beef Smokies Oscar Mayer	1	130	6	12	1	0	455	78	NA	*	3	8	*	*	4
Beef bologna Oscar Mayer	2 sl	150	5	13	1	0	478	68	NA	*	4	12	*	*	*
Beef franks Oscar Mayer	1	145	5	13	1	0	466	71	NA	2	5	18	*	*	3

Beef, Processed, cont'd.

Food	Serving	Calories	Protein g	Fat g	Carbo g	Fiber g	Sodium mg	Potassium mg	Vit A %rda	Vit B1 %rda (thiamin)	Vit B2 %rda (riboflavin)	Vit B3 %rda (niacin)	Vit C %rda	Calcium %rda	Iron %rda
Corned beef, jellied loaf Oscar Mayer	2 sl	90	13	4	0	0	572	50	NA	*	*	4	6	*	6
Corned hash	1 c	400	19	25	24	0	1520	440	NA	1	12	23	NA	3	24
Corned, canned	2 oz	123	15	7	0	0	595	NA	NA	0	8	10	NA	1	14
Dried, chipped	2 oz	116	19	3	0	0	2472	114	NA	3	11	11	0	1	16
Lean 'n Tasty Oscar Mayer	4 sl	160	12	12	0	0	808	152	NA	*	*	12	20	*	*

Chicken, Fresh

Food	Serving	Calories	Protein g	Fat g	Carbo g	Fiber g	Sodium mg	Potassium mg	Vit A %rda	Vit B1 %rda (thiamin)	Vit B2 %rda (riboflavin)	Vit B3 %rda (niacin)	Vit C %rda	Calcium %rda	Iron %rda
Breast, fried	½	160	26	5	1	0	NA	NA	1	3	10	58	NA	1	7
Broiled	4 oz	155	27	5	0	0	79	312	2	4	13	50	NA	1	11
Broiler, dark meat w/o skin	4 oz	232	31	11	0	0	105	272	2	6	15	37	0	2	8

Chicken, Fresh, cont'd.

Food	Serving	Calories	Protein g	Fat g	Carbo g	Fiber g	Sodium mg	Potassium mg	Vit A %rda	Vit B1 %rda (thiamin)	Vit B2 %rda (riboflavin)	Vit B3 %rda (niacin)	Vit C %rda	Calcium %rda	Iron %rda
Broiler, dark meat w/skin	4 oz	287 ●	29 ●	18 ○	0 ○	0 ○	99 ●	249 ●	5 ○	5 ○	14 ●	36 ●	0 ○	2 ○	9 ○
Broiler, light meat w/o skin	4 oz	196 ○	35 ●	5 ●	0 ○	0 ○	87 ●	280 ●	1 ○	5 ○	8 ○	70 ●	0 ○	2 ○	7 ○
Broiler, light meat w/skin	4 oz	252 ●	33 ●	12 ○	0 ○	0 ○	85 ●	257 ●	3 ●	5 ○	8 ○	63 ●	0 ○	2 ○	7 ○
Capons, roasted w/skin	4 oz	260 ●	33 ●	13 ○	0 ○	0 ○	56 ●	289 ●	2 ○	5 ○	11 ●	51 ●	0 ○	2 ○	9 ○
Drumstick, fried	1	88 ○	12 ●	4 ●	0 ○	0 ○	NA	NA	1 ○	2 ○	9 ○	14 ●	NA	1 ○	5 ○
Liver, simmered	4 oz	178 ●	27 ●	6 ●	0 ○	0 ○	58 ●	159 ○	371 ●	11 ●	117 ●	25 ●	29 ●	1 ○	53 ●
Roaster, dark meat w/o skin	4 oz	202 ●	26 ●	10 ○	0 ○	0 ○	108 ○	254 ○	1 ○	5 ○	13 ●	33 ●	0 ○	1 ○	8 ○
Roaster, light & dark, w/o skin	4 oz	189 ○	28 ●	8 ○	0 ○	0 ○	85 ●	260 ●	1 ○	5 ○	10 ●	45 ●	0 ○	1 ○	8 ○
Roaster, light & dark, w/skin	4 oz	253 ●	27 ●	15 ○	0 ○	0 ○	83 ●	239 ●	2 ○	4 ○	10 ●	42 ●	0 ○	1 ○	8 ○
Roaster, light meat w/o skin	4 oz	174 ●	31 ●	5 ●	0 ○	0 ○	58 ●	268 ●	1 ○	5 ○	6 ○	59 ●	0 ○	2 ○	7 ○

Chicken, Fresh, cont'd.

Food	Serving	Calories	Protein g	Fat g	Carbo g	Fiber g	Sodium mg	Potassium mg	Vit A %rda	Vit B1 %rda (thiamin)	Vit B2 %rda (riboflavin)	Vit B3 %rda (niacin)	Vit C %rda	Calcium %rda	Iron %rda
Thigh, fried	1	122	15	6	1	0	NA	NA	2	2	15	18	1	1	7
Wing, fried	1	82	9	5	1	0	NA	NA	2	1	5	11	0	0	3

Chicken, Processed

Food	Serving	Calories	Protein g	Fat g	Carbo g	Fiber g	Sodium mg	Potassium mg	Vit A %rda	Vit B1 %rda (thiamin)	Vit B2 %rda (riboflavin)	Vit B3 %rda (niacin)	Vit C %rda	Calcium %rda	Iron %rda
Canned chicken	2 oz	113	12	7	0	0	284	78	3	1	4	12	1	5	5
Chicken salad Carnation	2 oz	119	7	9	0	0	230	87	*	*	2	10	*	*	*

Cornish Hen, Duck & Goose

Food	Serving	Calories	Protein g	Fat g	Carbo g	Fiber g	Sodium mg	Potassium mg	Vit A %rda	Vit B1 %rda (thiamin)	Vit B2 %rda (riboflavin)	Vit B3 %rda (niacin)	Vit C %rda	Calcium %rda	Iron %rda
Cornish hen, w/skin	4 oz	257	28	14	0	0	NA	NA	2	4	36	51	3	4	31
Duck, roasted w/o skin	4 oz	228	27	13	0	0	74	286	2	20	31	29	0	1	17
Duck, roasted w/skin	4 oz	382	22	32	0	0	67	231	5	13	18	27	0	1	17

Cornish Hen, Duck & Goose, cont'd.

Food	Serving	Calories	Protein g	Fat g	Carbo g	Fiber g	Sodium mg	Potassium mg	Vit A %rda	Vit B1 %rda (thiamin)	Vit B2 %rda (riboflavin)	Vit B3 %rda (niacin)	Vit C %rda	Calcium %rda	Iron %rda
Goose, roasted w/o skin	4 oz	270	33	14	0	0	86	440	NA	7	26	23	0	2	18
Goose, roasted w/skin	4 oz	346	29	25	0	0	79	373	2	6	22	24	0	2	18

Fish and Shellfish

Food	Serving	Calories	Protein g	Fat g	Carbo g	Fiber g	Sodium mg	Potassium mg	Vit A %rda	Vit B1 %rda (thiamin)	Vit B2 %rda (riboflavin)	Vit B3 %rda (niacin)	Vit C %rda	Calcium %rda	Iron %rda
Bluefish, baked w/butter	4 oz	180	29	5	0	0	115	NA	1	8	6	11	NA	3	4
Caviar, sturgeon	2 tb	74	8	4	1	0	624	51	NA	1	7	NA	NA	8	18
Clams, canned	4 oz	60	9	3	0	0	NA	159	NA	1	7	6	NA	6	26
Clams, fried, 5 oz, Mrs Paul's	½	270	16	25	NA	0	675	NA	0	6	4	10	4	0	4
Cod, broiled w/butter	4 oz	192	32	6	0	0	460	124	5	7	7	18	NA	7	7
Cod, broiled w/o fats	4 oz	109	25	1	0	0	NA	NA	1	6	6	16	4	1	3
Cod, canned	1 c	119	27	0	0	0	NA	NA	NA	NA	6	NA	NA	NA	NA

Fish and Shellfish, cont'd.

Food	Serving	Calories	Protein g	Fat g	Carbo g	Fiber g	Sodium mg	Potassium mg	Vit A %rda	Vit B1 %rda (thiamin)	Vit B2 %rda (riboflavin)	Vit B3 %rda (niacin)	Vit C %rda	Calcium %rda	Iron %rda
Crabmeat, canned	1 c	135	24●	3●	0	0	149○	NA	NA	7○	6○	13●	NA	6○	6○
Crabmeat, cooked	1 c	144	27●	3●	1○	0	NA	NA	67●	17●	7○	22●	5○	7○	7○
Fillet light batter Mrs Paul's	2 pc	350	12●	18○	34●	NA	675○	NA	0○	10●	8●	10●	0○	4○	4○
Fillets, buttered Mrs Paul's	2 pc	310	16●	26●	2○	0	600○	NA	6○	10●	4○	20●	0○	0○	0○
Fillets, fried Mrs Paul's	2 pc	220	12●	9○	24●	NA	760○	NA	0○	10●	10●	15●	0○	4○	0○
Fish cakes Mrs Paul's	2 pc	210	10●	8○	23●	NA	NA	NA	0○	4○	6○	15●	0○	4○	0○
Fish sticks Mrs Paul's	4 pc	150	9●	5●	16●	NA	540○	NA	0○	4○	4○	10●	0○	2○	0○
Fish'n chips, light batter, 14 oz Mrs Paul's	½	370	16●	16●	45●	NA	1050○	NA	0○	15●	10●	60●	10○	10●	10●
Flounder w/lemon butter, 8.5 oz Mrs Paul's	½	150	11●	8○	9○	0	808○	NA	10○	8●	6○	25●	0○	4○	4○

Fish and Shellfish, cont'd.

Food	Serving	Calories	Protein g	Fat g	Carbo g	Fiber g	Sodium mg	Potassium mg	Vit A %rda	VitB1 %rda (thiamin)	VitB2 %rda (riboflavin)	VitB3 %rda (niacin)	Vit C %rda	Calcium %rda	Iron %rda
Flounder, baked w/butter	4 oz	228	34	9	0	0	268	664	NA	5	5	14	7	3	9
Haddock, breaded, fried	4 oz	187	23	7	7	NA	199	395	NA	3	5	18	5	5	7
Haddock, panfried	4 oz	188	22	6	0	0	200	396	NA	3	5	18	7	4	7
Lobster, cooked	1 c	138	27	2	0	0	305	261	NA	10	6	18	9	9	7
Mackerel, broiled w/butter	4 oz	268	25	18	0	0	NA	NA	12	11	19	44	1	1	7
Mackerel, canned	4 oz	204	24	11	0	0	NA	NA	1	2	22	50	NA	30	14
Oysters, canned	4 oz	103	12	3	6	0	NA	NA	7	9	NA	57	30	10	45
Oysters, raw	4 oz	76	10	2	4	0	84	136	NA	11	12	14	11	11	36
Perch fillet, fried	1	195	16	11	6	0	128	242	NA	7	6	8	3	3	6
Salmon, broiled	4 oz	208	31	8	0	0	132	504	4	13	5	56	NA	6	7
Salmon, pink, canned	4 oz	160	23	7	0	0	439	410	2	2	12	45	22	22	5

Fish and Shellfish, cont'd.

Food	Serving	Calories	Protein g	Fat g	Carbo g	Fiber g	Sodium mg	Potassium mg	Vit A %rda	Vit B1 %rda (thiamin)	Vit B2 %rda (riboflavin)	Vit B3 %rda (niacin)	Vit C %rda	Calcium %rda	Iron %rda
Salmon, red, canned	4 oz	194	23	11	0	0	593	391	5	3	11	42	NA	29	7
Salmon, smoked	4 oz	200	24	10	0	0	NA	NA	NA	NA	NA	NA	NA	2	NA
Sardines, oil-pack	4 oz	233	27	12	0	0	735	669	2	2	13	31	NA	50	19
Scallops, fried 7 oz, Mrs Paul's	½	210	12	8	24	NA	NA	NA	0	0	4	15	0	6	0
Scallops, light batter, 7 oz Mrs Paul's	½	200	12	8	21	NA	735	NA	10	10	10	20	0	2	4
Scallops, steamed	4 oz	127	26	2	0	0	301	540	NA	NA	NA	NA	NA	13	19
Seafood combo 9 oz, Mrs Paul's	1	510	20	22	57	0	2160	NA	25	10	40	10	15	15	15
Shad, baked w/butter	4 oz	228	26	13	0	0	88	428	11	16	48	NA	3	4	4
Shrimp, canned	4 oz	133	28	1	0	0	2607	138	1	3	11	NA	13	19	19
Shrimp, fried, 6 oz, Mrs Paul's	½	170	9	11	17	NA	480	NA	8	4	10	0	2	2	2

Fish and Shellfish, cont'd.

Food	Serving	Calories	Protein g	Fat g	Carbo g	Fiber g	Sodium mg	Potassium mg	Vit A %rda	Vit B1 %rda (thiamin)	Vit B2 %rda (riboflavin)	Vit B3 %rda (niacin)	Vit C %rda	Calcium %rda	Iron %rda
Sole, baked w/o fats	4 oz	105	24 ●	1 ●	0 ○	0 ○	NA	NA	1 ○	5 ○	4 ○	12 ●	NA	2 ○	6 ○
Tuna Helper, country dumpling, prepared	1/5	230	13 ●	6 ●	31 ●	NA	1020 ○	NA	* ○	20 ●	10 ●	30 ●	* ○	4 ○	10 ●
Tuna Helper, creamy noodle, prepared	1/5	280	13 ●	11 ○	31 ●	NA	880 ○	NA	6 ○	20 ●	10 ●	30 ●	* ○	2 ○	10 ●
Tuna Helper, noodles almondine, prepared	1/5	240	6 ●	12 ○	27 ●	NA	835 ○	NA	6 ○	15 ●	15 ●	8 ○	* ○	8 ○	6 ○
Tuna salad Carnation	1/4 cn	98	6 ●	7 ●	3 ○	0 ○	268 ●	105 ○	* ○	* ○	* ○	14 ●	* ○	* ○	2 ○
Tuna, canned, water-pack	4 oz	144	32 ●	1 ●	0 ○	0 ○	450 ●	316 ●	NA	NA	7 ○	75 ●	NA	2 ○	10 ●
Tuna, canned, water pack, low sodium	4 oz	144	32 ●	1 ●	0 ○	0 ○	46 ●	316 ●	NA	NA	7 ○	75 ●	NA	2 ○	10 ●
Tuna, oil-pack	4 oz	227	32 ●	9 ●	0 ○	0 ○	403 ○	NA	2 ○	4 ○	8 ○	67 ●	NA	1 ○	12 ●
Whitefish, smoked	4 oz	176	24 ●	8 ○	0 ○	NA	NA	NA	NA	NA	NA	NA	NA ○	3 ○	NA

Lamb

Food	Serving	Calories	Protein g	Fat g	Carbo g	Fiber g	Sodium mg	Potassium mg	Vit A % rda	Vit B1 % rda (thiamin)	Vit B2 % rda (riboflavin)	Vit B3 % rda (niacin)	Vit C % rda	Calcium % rda	Iron % rda
Leg roast, untrimmed	4 oz	313	29	21	0	0	70	321	NA	12	18	31	NA	1	10
Leg roast, trimmed	4 oz	208	32	8	0	0	77	363	NA	13	20	35	NA	1	12
Loin chop, broiled, trimmed	4 oz	213	32	9	0	0	78	358	NA	11	19	35	NA	1	13
Loin chop, broiled, untrimmed	4 oz	407	25	33	0	0	61	280	NA	9	15	28	NA	1	8
Rib chop, trimmed	4 oz	240	32	12	0	0	56	348	NA	12	18	34	NA	1	12
Rib chop, untrimmed	4 oz	465	23	41	0	0	76	258	NA	9	14	26	NA	1	7
Shoulder roast, trimmed	4 oz	226	30	10	0	0	75	336	NA	12	18	32	NA	1	10
Shoulder roast, untrimmed	4 oz	380	24	31	0	0	70	275	NA	10	16	27	NA	1	7

Meat Substitutes

Food	Serving	Calories	Protein g	Fat g	Carbo g	Fiber g	Sodium mg	Potassium mg	Vit A %rda	Vit B1 %rda (thiamin)	Vit B2 %rda (riboflavin)	Vit B3 %rda (niacin)	Vit C %rda	Calcium %rda	Iron %rda
Breakfast link Morningstar	3	186	16	14	1	0	598	100	*	53	17	28	*	3	19
Breakfast patty Morningstar	2	221	16	14	6	0	818	115	*	87	24	44	*	5	24
Breakfast strip Morningstar	4	152	4	1	1	0	396	51	*	8	8	8	*	*	4
Grillers Morningstar	1	189	16	12	5	NA	284	105	*	25	15	25	*	*	20
Luncheon slice Morningstar	2 sl	49	6	2	3	NA	675	82	*	33	16	15	*	2	10

Pork, Fresh

Food	Serving	Calories	Protein g	Fat g	Carbo g	Fiber g	Sodium mg	Potassium mg	Vit A %rda	Vit B1 %rda (thiamin)	Vit B2 %rda (riboflavin)	Vit B3 %rda (niacin)	Vit C %rda	Calcium %rda	Iron %rda
Loin chop, untrimmed	4 oz	452	28	37	0	0	68	320	0	74	19	33	NA	1	22
Loin chop, trimmed	4 oz	300	34	18	0	0	82	384	0	84	21	38	NA	1	24
Roast, trimmed	4 oz	292	33	17	0	0	78	373	0	81	21	37	NA	2	24
Roast, untrimmed	4 oz	413	28	32	0	0	68	311	0	69	17	32	NA	1	20

Pork, Processed

Food	Serving	Calories	Protein g	Fat g	Carbo g	Fiber g	Sodium mg	Potassium mg	Vit A %rda	Vit B1 %rda (thiamin)	Vit B2 %rda (riboflavin)	Vit B3 %rda (niacin)	Vit C %rda	Calcium %rda	Iron %rda
Bacon	4 sl	170	8 ●	16 ○	0 ○	0 ○	587 ○	70 ○	11 ●	6 ○	8 ○	NA	0 ○	0 ○	6 ○
Bologna, Oscar Mayer	2 sl	150	5 ●	14 ○	1 ○	0 ○	482 ○	72 ○	6 ○	* ○	4 ○	12 ○	* ○	* ○	* ○
Braunschweiger, Oscar Mayer	2 sl	190	7 ●	17 ○	2 ○	NA	660 ○	102 ○	8 ○	50 ●	22 ●	8 ○	* ○	8 ○	30 ●
Canadian bacon, Oscar Mayer	2 sl	80	12 ●	4 ●	0 ○	0 ○	786 ●	168 ○	26 ●	4 ○	14 ●	24 ●	* ○	* ○	* ○
Cheese Smokies, Oscar Mayer	1	140	6 ●	13 ○	0 ○	NA	450 ○	85 ○	7 ○	4 ○	4 ○	12 ○	2 ○	2 ○	2 ○
Franks	1	170	7 ●	15 ○	1 ○	0 ○	627 ○	NA	5 ○	6 ○	6 ○	NA	0 ○	0 ○	4 ○
Ham roast, untrimmed	4 oz	327	24 ●	25 ●	0 ○	0 ○	1485 ●	265 ●	36 ●	12 ●	21 ●	NA	1 ○	1 ●	16 ●
Ham salad, Carnation	¼ cn	107	8 ●	8 ○	4 ○	0 ○	333 ○	144 ○	11 ●	4 ○	7 ○	* ○	* ○	6 ○	6 ○
Ham steak Jubilee, Oscar Mayer	2 sl	140	22 ●	6 ●	0 ○	0 ○	1482 ●	378 ●	62 ●	14 ●	28 ●	62 ●	* ○	* ○	6 ○
Ham, cooked, Oscar Mayer	2 sl	50	8 ●	2 ●	0 ○	NA	564 ○	146 ○	26 ●	4 ○	10 ●	16 ○	* ○	1 ○	6 ○
Ham, luncheon, thin-slice	2 sl	130	10 ○	10 ○	0 ○	0 ○	NA	NA	16 ○	5 ○	7 ○	NA	1 ○	1 ○	9 ○

Pork, Processed, cont'd.

Food	Serving	Calories	Protein g	Fat g	Carbo g	Fiber g	Sodium mg	Potassium mg	Vit A %rda	Vit B1 %rda (thiamin)	Vit B2 %rda (riboflavin)	Vit B3 %rda (niacin)	Vit C %rda	Calcium %rda	Iron %rda
Lean 'n Tasty Oscar Mayer	4 sl	180	12	14	0	0	880	NA	20	8	8	28	*	*	*
Little Friers Oscar Mayer	2	160	6	15	0	0	446	NA	12	4	8	*	*	*	*
Liver cheese Oscar Mayer	2 sl	230	11	20	1	NA	912	NA	10	98	42	*	*	50	*
Luncheon meat Oscar Mayer	2 sl	190	7	18	1	0	716	NA	10	4	8	12	*	*	*
Peppered loaf Oscar Mayer	2 sl	80	10	4	3	0	798	NA	14	3	8	20	*	*	*
Picnic loaf Oscar Mayer	2 sl	130	8	9	3	0	640	NA	14	6	6	14	*	8	*
Salami	2 oz	180	10	14	0	0	595	NA	9	8	12	NA	*	*	*
Salami for beer Oscar Mayer	2 sl	110	6	9	1	0	564	NA	16	4	6	22	1	*	*
Sandwich spread Oscar Mayer	2 oz	130	4	10	6	NA	550	NA	6	4	4	*	*	*	*
Sausage links	1	60	2	6	0	0	168	0	7	2	3	NA	0	2	0

Pork, Processed, cont'd.

Food	Serving	Calories	Protein g	Fat g	Carbo g	Fiber g	Sodium mg	Potassium mg	Vit A %rda	Vit B1 %rda (thiamin)	Vit B2 %rda (riboflavin)	Vit B3 %rda (niacin)	Vit C %rda	Calcium %rda	Iron %rda
Wieners Oscar Mayer	1	145	5	14	1	0	459	73	6	2	2	19	*	2	2
Wieners, w/cheese Oscar Mayer	1	145	5	14	1	0	510	56	5	3	3	15	2	2	2

Turkey, Fresh

Food	Serving	Calories	Protein g	Fat g	Carbo g	Fiber g	Sodium mg	Potassium mg	Vit A %rda	Vit B1 %rda (thiamin)	Vit B2 %rda (riboflavin)	Vit B3 %rda (niacin)	Vit C %rda	Calcium %rda	Iron %rda
Dark meat w/o skin	4 oz	233	35	9	0	0	112	451	NA	3	16	24	NA	NA	15
Light & dark meat w/o skin, chopped	1 c	265	44	9	0	0	111	514	NA	5	15	54	NA	1	14
Light & dark meat, w/o skin	4 oz	193	33	6	0	0	79	338	0	5	12	31	0	3	11
Light meat w/o skin	4 oz	200	37	4	0	0	59	465	NA	4	9	63	NA	NA	7

Turkey, Processed

Food	Serving	Calories	Protein g	Fat g	Carbo g	Fiber g	Sodium mg	Potassium mg	Vit A %rda	Vit B1 %rda (thiamin)	Vit B2 %rda (riboflavin)	Vit B3 %rda (niacin)	Vit C %rda	Calcium %rda	Iron %rda
Bologna, Louis Rich	2 sl	120	7 ●	9 ○	1 ○	0 ○	444 ○	106 ○	* ○	4 ○	10 ○	NA	4 ○	4 ○	4 ○
Breast, oven-roasted, Louis Rich	2 sl	60	12 ●	2 ●	0 ○	0 ○	380 ○	126 ○	* ○	4 ○	20 ●	NA	* ○	* ○	4 ○
Franks, Louis Rich	1	100	6 ○	8 ○	1 ○	0 ○	472 ○	72 ○	1 ○	4 ○	8 ○	NA	5 ○	* ○	4 ○
Ham, Louis Rich	2 sl	70	11 ●	2 ●	0 ○	0 ○	576 ○	174 ○	2 ○	8 ○	16 ●	NA	* ○	4 ○	4 ○
Pastrami, Louis Rich	2 sl	70	11 ●	3 ●	0 ○	0 ○	556 ○	174 ○	* ○	8 ○	14 ●	NA	* ○	4 ○	4 ○
Salami, Louis Rich	2 sl	100	9 ●	7 ●	1 ○	0 ○	502 ○	126 ○	* ○	8 ○	12 ●	NA	* ○	* ○	4 ○
Turkey salad, Carnation	¼ cn	109	8 ●	8 ○	3 ○	0 ○	245 ●	103 ●	* ○	* ○	11 ●	* ○	* ○	* ○	* ○

Veal

Food	Serving	Calories	Protein g	Fat g	Carbo g	Fiber g	Sodium mg	Potassium mg	Vit A %rda	Vit B1 %rda (thiamin)	Vit B2 %rda (riboflavin)	Vit B3 %rda (niacin)	Vit C %rda	Calcium %rda	Iron %rda
Calf liver, fried	4 oz	296 ●	33 ●	15 ○	5 ○	0 ○	133 ●	513 ●	741 ●	18 ●	278 ●	93 ●	69 ●	2 ○	90 ●
Cubes, untrimmed	4 oz	267 ●	32 ●	15 ○	0 ○	0 ○	56 ●	253 ●	NA	7 ○	19 ●	36 ●	NA	1 ○	22 ●

Veal, cont'd.

Food	Serving	Calories	Protein g	Fat g	Carbo g	Fiber g	Sodium mg	Potassium mg	Vit A %rda	Vit B1 %rda (thiamin)	Vit B2 %rda (riboflavin)	Vit B3 %rda (niacin)	Vit C %rda	Calcium %rda	Iron %rda
Cutlet, broiled	4 oz	247 ●	31 ●	12 ○	0 ○	0 ○	75 ●	344 ●	NA	5 ○	16 ●	31 ●	NA	1 ○	20 ●
Loin chop, trimmed	4 oz	235	39 ●	8 ○	0 ○	0 ○	74 ●	539 ●	0 ○	16 ●	22 ●	41 ●	0 ○	2 ○	27 ●
Loin chop, untrimmed	4 oz	478	26 ●	41 ○	0 ○	0 ○	50 ●	357 ●	0 ○	10 ●	14 ●	27 ●	0 ○	1 ○	18 ●
Rib chop, trimmed	4 oz	244	39 ●	10 ○	0 ○	0 ○	68 ●	643 ●	0 ○	16 ●	22 ●	41 ●	0 ○	2 ○	27 ●
Rib chop, untrimmed	4 oz	361	31 ●	25 ○	0 ○	0 ○	56 ●	529 ●	0 ○	12 ●	18 ●	33 ●	0 ○	2 ○	22 ●
Rib roast, untrimmed	4 oz	307	31 ●	19 ○	0 ○	0 ○	91 ●	345 ●	NA	10 ●	20 ●	44 ●	NA	1 ○	22 ●
Rump roast, trimmed	4 oz	173	35 ●	2 ●	0 ○	0 ○	147 ●	1158 ○	0 ○	28 ●	29 ●	99 ●	0 ○	2 ○	25 ●
Rump roast, untrimmed	4 oz	193	34 ●	5 ●	0 ○	0 ○	83 ●	562 ●	0 ○	11 ●	13 ●	45 ●	0 ○	1 ○	24 ●
Scallopini	4 oz	199	20 ●	11 ○	3 ○	0 ○	918 ○	385 ●	2 ○	3 ○	17 ●	51 ●	* ○	11 ●	12 ●

Sweets & Snacks
Cakes, Prepared

Food	Serving	Calories	Protein g	Fat g	Carbo g	Fiber g	Sodium mg	Potassium mg	Vit A %rda	Vit B1 %rda (thiamin)	Vit B2 %rda (riboflavin)	Vit B3 %rda (niacin)	Vit C %rda	Calcium %rda	Iron %rda
Angel food, chocolate, Betty Crocker	1/2	140	3	0	32	NA	275	NA	*	*	6	*	*	*	*
Angel food, one-step, Betty Crocker	1/2	140	3	0	32	NA	250	NA	*	*	6	*	4	*	*
Angel food, raspberry, Pillsbury	1/2	140	3	0	33	NA	330	0	0	2	6	0	2	0	0
Angel food, strawberry, Betty Crocker	1/2	150	3	0	34	NA	270	*	*	*	4	*	4	4	*
Angel food, traditional, Betty Crocker	1/2	130	3	0	30	NA	140	*	*	*	6	*	4	4	*
Apple walnut w/ cream cheese icing, Pepperidge Farm	1/6	150	1	8	18	NA	140	NA	NA	NA	NA	NA	NA	NA	NA
Banana, Pillsbury	1/12	260	3	11	36	NA	305	2	8	6	6	0	4	4	4
Boston cream, Pepperidge Farm	1/4	290	3	14	39	NA	190	NA	NA	NA	NA	NA	NA	NA	NA

Cakes, Prepared, cont'd.

Food	Serving	Calories	Protein g	Fat g	Carbo g	Fiber g	Sodium mg	Potassium mg	Vit A %rda	Vit B1 %rda (thiamin)	Vit B2 %rda (riboflavin)	Vit B3 %rda (niacin)	Vit C %rda	Calcium %rda	Iron %rda
Brownie mix, fudge Betty Crocker	1/24	150	1	6	22	NA	100	*	2	2	2	*	*	4	4
Brownie, double fudge, 16 oz Duncan Hines	1/16	140	2	5	21	NA	105	*	2	2	2	*	*	2	2
Bundt, chocolate macaroon Pillsbury	1/16	250	3	11	35	NA	315	2	8	6	4	0	0	4	4
Bundt, lemon-blueberry Pillsbury	1/16	200	3	8	28	NA	270	4	6	6	2	0	4	6	6
Bundt, triple fudge Pillsbury	1/16	210	3	9	30	NA	330	4	6	4	2	0	4	6	6
Bundt, tunnel of lemon Pillsbury	1/16	270	2	10	43	NA	290	2	6	6	2	0	6	4	4
Bundt, fudge nut Pillsbury	1/16	220	3	9	31	NA	290	4	4	4	2	0	2	6	6
Carrot 'n spice Pillsbury	1/12	260	3	11	35	NA	335	25	8	6	4	4	4	6	6

Cakes, Prepared, cont'd.

Food	Serving	Calories	Protein g	Fat g	Carbo g	Fiber g	Sodium mg	Potassium mg	Vit A %rda	Vit B1 %rda (thiamin)	Vit B2 %rda (riboflavin)	Vit B3 %rda (niacin)	Vit C %rda	Calcium %rda	Iron %rda
Carrot w/cream cheese icing Pepperidge Farm	1/8	140	1	8	17	NA	145	NA	NA	NA	NA	NA	NA	NA	NA
Cheesecake, Jell-O	1/8	300	6	14	38	NA	365	240	8	8	15	2	*	20	2
Choco-Dile	1 pc	250	2	11	37	NA	225	NA	0	4	4	0	0	2	4
Chocolate Junior	1 pc	354	4	12	56	NA	292	NA	NA	NA	NA	NA	NA	NA	NA
Chocolate fudge Pepperidge Farm	1/10	190	1	10	23	NA	140	NA	NA	NA	NA	NA	NA	NA	NA
Chocolate mint Pillsbury	1/12	250	4	12	33	NA	375	NA	2	8	6	4	0	10	6
Chocolate, sour cream Duncan Hines	1/12	200	3	6	34	NA	330	NA	*	*	4	6	*	10	6
Coconut Pepperidge Farm	1/10	180	1	9	25	NA	120	NA	NA	NA	NA	NA	NA	NA	NA
Coconut Junior	1 pc	330	4	7	60	NA	327	NA	NA	NA	NA	NA	NA	NA	NA

Cakes, Prepared, cont'd.

Food	Serving	Calories	Protein g	Fat g	Carbo g	Fiber g	Sodium mg	Potassium mg	Vit A %rda	Vit B1 %rda (thiamin)	Vit B2 %rda (riboflavin)	Vit B3 %rda (niacin)	Vit C %rda	Calcium %rda	Iron %rda
Coffeecake mix Aunt Jemima	1/6	170	3	5	29	NA	270	45	*	6	4	*	6	2	2
Coffeecake, butter pecan Pillsbury	1/6	310	4	15	39	NA	335	NA	8	10	8	0	4	4	4
Coffeecake, sour cream Pillsbury	1/6	270	4	12	35	NA	235	NA	4	8	8	0	4	4	4
Creamie, chocolate	1 pc	195	2	9	25	NA	114	NA	NA	NA	NA	NA	NA	NA	NA
Creamie, vanilla	1 pc	209	1	10	28	NA	126	NA	NA	NA	NA	NA	NA	NA	NA
Cupcake, chocolate Tastykake	1 pc	117	2	3	20	NA	172	NA	NA	NA	NA	NA	NA	NA	NA
Cupcake, chocolate, cream-filled Tastykake	1 pc	124	2	3	21	NA	161	NA	NA	NA	NA	NA	NA	NA	NA
Cupcake, orange Hostess	1 pc	150	1	4	27	NA	150	0	0	4	2	0	2	2	2
Cupcake, yellow w/icing	1	130	2	5	21	NA	121	42	1	3	4	*	5	2	2

Cakes, Prepared, cont'd.

Food	Serving	Calories	Protein g	Fat g	Carbo g	Fiber g	Sodium mg	Potassium mg	Vit A %rda	Vit B1 %rda (thiamin)	Vit B2 %rda (riboflavin)	Vit B3 %rda (niacin)	Vit C %rda	Calcium %rda	Iron %rda
Cupcake, yellow w/o icing	1	90	1	3●	14	NA	113●	21	1	3	3	2	*	4	2
Devil's food Pillsbury	1/12	250	2	11	35	NA	410	NA	0	2	2	2	0	10●	4
Ding Dongs	1 pc	170	1	10	21	NA	95●	NA	0	0	2	0	0	2	2
Donut, old fashioned Hostess	1 pc	170	2	10	20	NA	150●	NA	0	6	4	4	0	2	2
Donut, powdered sugar Hostess	1 pc	110	1	6●	15	NA	110●	NA	0	2	2	2	0	2	2
Donut, cinnamon Hostess	1 pc	110	1	6●	15	NA	110●	NA	0	2	2	2	0	2	2
Donut, glazed	1	205	3	11	22	NA	117●	34	1	7	6	4	0	2	3
Donut, krunch Hostess	1 pc	100	1	4●	16	NA	105●	NA	0	2	2	2	0	2	2
Donut, plain	1	100	1	5●	13	NA	125●	23	0	3	3	*	*	1	2
Fruitcake	1 sl	55	1	2●	9	NA	29●	74	0	1	1	*	*	1	2

Cakes, Prepared, cont'd.

Food	Serving	Calories	Protein g	Fat g	Carbo g	Fiber g	Sodium mg	Potassium mg	Vit A %rda	Vit B1 %rda (thiamin)	Vit B2 %rda (riboflavin)	Vit B3 %rda (niacin)	Vit C %rda	Calcium %rda	Iron %rda
Fudge, butter recipe Duncan Hines	1/12	270	4	13	34	NA	350	NA	6	2	8	*	2	2	6
German chocolate Pepperidge Farm	1/10	180	1	10	23	NA	170	NA	NA	NA	NA	NA	NA	NA	NA
Gingerbread Pillsbury	1/9	190	2	4	36	NA	340	NA	0	8	6	0	4	4	8
Golden layer Pepperidge Farm	1/10	180	1	9	24	NA	115	NA	NA	NA	NA	NA	NA	NA	NA
Golden, butter recipe Duncan Hines	1/12	270	3	13	36	NA	270	NA	4	4	6	*	4	4	4
Ho Hos	1 pc	120	1	6	17	NA	80	NA	0	0	2	0	2	2	2
Kandy Kake, chocolate	1 pc	95	1	4	12	NA	64	NA	NA	NA	NA	NA	NA	NA	NA
Kandy Kake, peanut butter	1 pc	105	2	6	11	NA	48	NA	NA	NA	NA	NA	NA	NA	NA
Koffee Kake	1 pc	329	4	12	49	NA	314	NA	NA	NA	NA	NA	NA	NA	NA

Cakes, Prepared, cont'd.

Food	Serving	Calories	Protein g	Fat g	Carbo g	Fiber g	Sodium mg	Potassium mg	Vit A %rda	Vit B1 %rda (thiamin)	Vit B2 %rda (riboflavin)	Vit B3 %rda (niacin)	Vit C %rda	Calcium %rda	Iron %rda
Krimpet, butterscotch Tastykake	1 pc	117	1○	3●	20○	NA	95●	NA	NA	NA	NA	NA	NA	NA	NA
Krimpet, jelly Tastykake	1 pc	98	1○	2●	19○	NA	104●	NA	NA	NA	NA	NA	NA	NA	NA
Layer, yellow, iced	1 pc	235	3○	8○	40○	NA	242●	75○	2○	5○	6○	4○	*○	6○	4○
Lemon chiffon Betty Crocker	1/6	190	4●	4○	35○	NA	190●	NA	*○	6○	8○	2○	*○	2○	4○
Lemon coconut Pepperidge Farm	1/4	280	2○	13●	38○	NA	220●	NA	NA	NA	NA	NA	NA	NA	NA
Moist & Easy, double chocolate chip	1/9	180	3○	5●	32○	NA	340○	NA	*○	*○	4○	4○	*○	6○	6○
Pound, from mix Dromedary	1/12	210	3○	9○	29○	NA	NA○	NA	2○	6○	4○	2○	*○	2	2
Pudding cake, chocolate Betty Crocker	1/6	230	2○	5●	45○	NA	255●	NA	2○	4○	4○	2○	*○	4○	6○
Pudding cake, lemon Betty Crocker	1/6	230	2○	5●	45○	NA	270●	NA	2○	4○	4○	2○	*○	2○	2○

Cakes, Prepared, cont'd.

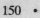

Food	Serving	Calories	Protein g	Fat g	Carbo g	Fiber g	Sodium mg	Potassium mg	Vit A %rda	Vit B1 %rda (thiamin)	Vit B2 %rda (riboflavin)	Vit B3 %rda (niacin)	Vit C %rda	Calcium %rda	Iron %rda
Quickbread, apricot nut Pillsbury	1/12	160	2	4	27	NA	150	NA	6	8	4	0	0	0	6
Quickbread, cherry nut Pillsbury	1/12	170	2	5	30	NA	150	NA	0	10	4	0	0	0	4
Quickbread, cranberry Pillsbury	1/12	160	2	4	28	NA	150	NA	0	8	4	0	0	0	4
Snackin' Cake, German chocolate	1/9	180	2	6	30	NA	255	NA	*	6	4	*	6	6	4
Snackin' Cake, banana walnut	1/9	190	2	6	31	NA	260	NA	*	6	4	*	4	4	2
Snackin' Cake, carrot nut	1/9	180	2	6	30	NA	240	NA	4	6	4	*	8	8	4
Snackin' Cake, golden chocolate chip	1/9	190	2	5	34	NA	255	NA	*	6	2	*	6	6	4
Sno Ball	1 pc	140	1	4	25	NA	165	NA	0	0	2	0	2	2	2
Sponge	1 pc	195	5	4	36	NA	110	57	6	6	3	*	2	2	6

Cakes, Prepared, cont'd.

Food	Serving	Calories	Protein g	Fat g	Carbo g	Fiber g	Sodium mg	Potassium mg	Vit A %rda	Vit B1 %rda (thiamin)	Vit B2 %rda (riboflavin)	Vit B3 %rda (niacin)	Vit C %rda	Calcium %rda	Iron %rda
Stir 'n Frost, lemon	1/6	230	2	7	39	NA	210	NA	*	6	4	2	*	2	2
Stir 'n Frost, spice	1/6	270	2	8	47	NA	305	NA	*	8	4	4	*	2	4
Stir 'n Frost, white	1/6	220	2	7	38	NA	235	NA	*	4	2	4	*	4	2
Stir 'n Frost, yellow	1/6	220	2	7	38	NA	210	NA	*	4	2	2	*	2	2
Stir 'n Streusel, cinnamon	1/6	240	3	7	42	NA	230	NA	*	8	4	6	*	*	4
Strawberry cream Pepperidge Farm	1/12	190	1	8	27	NA	145	NA	NA	NA	NA	NA	NA	NA	NA
Strawberry supreme Duncan Hines	1/12	200	3	5	35	NA	240	NA	*	4	4	4	*	6	4
Supermoist, Butter Brickle	1/12	260	3	11	37	NA	255	NA	*	6	6	4	*	6	4
Supermoist, butter pecan	1/12	250	3	11	35	NA	250	NA	*	6	4	4	*	4	4
Supermoist, chocolate fudge	1/12	250	3	11	35	NA	450	NA	*	6	4	4	*	6	6
Supermoist, carrot	1/12	250	3	11	35	NA	255	NA	*	6	4	4	*	4	4

Cakes, Prepared, cont'd.

Food	Serving	Calories	Protein g	Fat g	Carbo g	Fiber g	Sodium mg	Potassium mg	Vit A %rda	Vit B1 %rda (thiamin)	Vit B2 %rda (riboflavin)	Vit B3 %rda (niacin)	Vit C %rda	Calcium %rda	Iron %rda
Supermoist, marble	1/12	270	3	11	40	NA	280	NA	*	6	6	4	6	6	6
Supermoist, orange	1/12	260	3	11	36	NA	280	NA	*	6	4	4	6	6	4
Suzy Q's, banana	1 pc	240	2	9	38	NA	195	NA	0	6	6	4	4	4	4
Suzy Q's, chocolate	1 pc	240	1	9	36	NA	310	NA	0	0	2	2	2	2	4
Tiger Tail	2 pc	430	4	13	76	NA	480	NA	2	10	10	6	6	6	10
Twinkies	1 pc	140	1	4	26	NA	190	NA	0	4	4	2	2	2	4
Upside-down cake, pineapple Betty Crocker	1/9	270	2	10	43	NA	215	NA	4	4	4	2	4	4	2
Vienna dream bar Betty Crocker	1/24	90	1	5	10	NA	65	NA	*	2	*	*	*	*	*
Walnut Pepperidge Farm	1/4	300	2	17	33	NA	200	NA	NA	NA	NA	NA	NA	*	*

Candy

Food	Serving	Calories	Protein g	Fat g	Carbo g	Fiber g	Sodium mg	Potassium mg	Vit A %rda	Vit B1 %rda (thiamin)	Vit B2 %rda (riboflavin)	Vit B3 %rda (niacin)	Vit C %rda	Calcium % rda	Iron % rda
$100,000, 1.5-oz bar	1	200	2	8	31	NA	75	70	*	*	4	*	4	*	*
3 Musketeers, 2.3-oz bar	1	280	2	8	49	0	135	NA	*	*	4	*	4	2	2
Almond Joy, 1.6-oz bar	1	242	3	13	30	NA	NA	NA	*	*	*	NA	3	7	7
Baby Ruth 1.8-oz bar	1	260	6	11	31	NA	100	150	*	*	6	*	2	2	2
Butterfinger 1.6-oz bar	1	220	4	10	28	NA	70	100	*	*	4	*	2	4	4
Caramello, 1.2-oz bar	1	173	1	10	20	0	NA	NA	*	*	8	NA	7	4	4
Caramels	1 oz	115	1	3	22	0	74	*	*	1	3	1	4	2	2
Chocolate morsels	¼ c	215	2	15	24	0	1	138	*	*	2	1	1	6	6
Chocolate, milk	1 oz	145	2	9	16	0	28	109	*	1	6	1	7	2	2
Fudge, chocolate	1 oz	115	1	3	21	0	54	42	*	1	2	1	2	2	2
Gum drops	1 oz	100	0	0	25	0	10	1	0	0	*	0	0	1	1

Candy, cont'd.

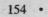

Food	Serving	Calories	Protein g	Fat g	Carbo g	Fiber g	Sodium mg	Potassium mg	Vit A %rda	Vit B1 %rda (thiamin)	Vit B2 %rda (riboflavin)	Vit B3 %rda (niacin)	Vit C %rda	Calcium %rda	Iron %rda
Hard	1 oz	110	0	0	28	0	9	1	0	0	0	0	1	1	3
Kisses, Hershey	6	150	2	9	16	0	25	115	*	*	*	*	6	6	2
Kit Kat, 1.1-oz bar	1	160	2	8	19	NA	30	95	*	4	*	*	6	6	2
Krackel, 1.2-oz bar	1	160	2	10	17	NA	30	120	*	4	*	*	6	6	2
M&M's, plain, 1.7-oz pk	1	240	3	10	33	NA	41	NA	*	4	6	*	8	8	4
M&M's, peanut, 1.7-oz pk	1	240	5	12	28	NA	29	NA	*	8	2	6	4	4	2
Mars bar, 1.7 oz	1	230	4	10	29	NA	71	NA	*	*	*	*	6	6	2
Marshmallows	1 oz	90	1	0	23	0	11	2	0	0	0	0	1	3	3
Milk chocolate w/almonds, 1-oz bar Hershey	1	160	3	10	16	NA	25	130	*	6	6	*	6	6	2
Milky Way, 2.1-oz bar	1	260	3	9	43	0	119	NA	*	6	*	*	6	2	2

Candy, cont'd.

Food	Serving	Calories	Protein g	Fat g	Carbo g	Fiber g	Sodium mg	Potassium mg	Vit A %rda	Vit B1 %rda (thiamin)	Vit B2 %rda (riboflavin)	Vit B3 %rda (niacin)	Vit C %rda	Calcium %rda	Iron %rda
Mints, plain	1 oz	105	0	1	25	0	56	1	0	*	*	0	0	2	2
Mounds, 1.6-oz bar	1	235	2	11	32	NA	NA	NA	*	*	*	NA	*	9	9
Mr. Goodbar, 1.3 oz	1	200	5	12	18	NA	20	165	2	6	10	*	6	4	4
Nestle Crunch 1-oz bar	1	150	2	8	18	NA	45	100	*	4	*	*	4	*	*
Peanut brittle Kraft	1 oz	140	3	5	20	NA	145	NA	2	*	8	*	*	*	*
Peppermint pattie 1.3 oz, York	1	161	1	3	33	0	NA	NA	*	*	*	NA	*	3	3
Powerhouse, 2-oz bar	1	262	5	10	38	NA	NA	NA	*	6	NA	NA	*	21	2
Reese's cups, 1.2-oz pk	1	180	4	11	17	NA	110	135	*	4	8	*	2	2	2
Rolo	5 pc	140	1	6	19	0	65	75	4	*	*	*	8	2	2
Snickers, 2-oz bar	1	270	6	13	33	NA	139	NA	*	4	8	*	6	2	2
Special dark chocolate, 1-oz bar	1	160	1	9	19	0	1	100	2	2	2	*	*	2	2

Candy, cont'd.

Food	Serving	Calories	Protein g	Fat g	Carbo g	Fiber g	Sodium mg	Potassium mg	Vit A %rda	Vit B1 %rda (thiamin)	Vit B2 %rda (riboflavin)	Vit B3 %rda (niacin)	Vit C %rda	Calcium %rda	Iron %rda
Starburst, 2-oz pk	1	240	0	5	49	0	26	NA	*	*	*	*	*	*	*
Summit, 1.5-oz pk	½	110	2	7	12	NA	30	NA	*	2	2	2	*	2	*
Toffee, Kraft	1 pc	30	0	1	5	NA	20	NA	*	*	*	*	*	*	*
Twix, 1.7-oz pk	½	130	3	7	14	NA	NA	NA	*	2	4	4	*	2	2
Whatchamacallit 1-oz bar	1	170	3	10	18	NA	70	100	*	4	4	4	*	4	*

Cookies (approx. 1 oz)

Food	Serving	Calories	Protein g	Fat g	Carbo g	Fiber g	Sodium mg	Potassium mg	Vit A %rda	Vit B1 %rda (thiamin)	Vit B2 %rda (riboflavin)	Vit B3 %rda (niacin)	Vit C %rda	Calcium %rda	Iron %rda
Animal, Barnum's	11	130	2	4	21	NA	NA	NA	*	4	6	4	*	4	4
Biscos sugar wafers	8	150	1	7	21	NA	50	NA	*	2	2	2	*	*	2
Bordeaux	4	146	1	7	21	NA	93	NA	NA	NA	NA	NA	NA	NA	NA
Brown edge wafers	5	140	1	6	21	NA	90	NA	*	6	2	4	*	*	2

Cookies (approx. 1 oz), cont'd.

Food	Serving	Calories	Protein g	Fat g	Carbo g	Fiber g	Sodium mg	Potassium mg	Vit A %rda	Vit B1 %rda (thiamin)	Vit B2 %rda (riboflavin)	Vit B3 %rda (niacin)	Vit C %rda	Calcium %rda	Iron %rda
Brownies w/nuts	1	85	1	4	13	NA	43	34	0	1	1	1	*	1	2
Brussels Mint	2	133	1	7	17	NA	80	NA	NA	NA	NA	NA	NA	NA	NA
Cappucino	3	160	1	9	18	NA	60	NA	NA	NA	NA	NA	NA	NA	NA
Capri	2	160	1	9	20	NA	90	NA	NA	NA	NA	NA	NA	NA	NA
Chessman	3	130	1	6	18	NA	80	NA	NA	NA	NA	NA	NA	NA	NA
Chips Ahoy!	3	160	2	7	21	NA	120	NA	4	4	4	4	*	4	4
Chocolate chip snaps Nabisco	6	120	2	4	20	NA	97	NA	4	4	4	2	*	2	2
Chocolate chip, slice 'n bake Pillsbury	3	160	1	8	22	NA	125	NA	4	4	4	4	0	0	0
Chocolate snaps Nabisco	8	130	2	4	22	NA	171	NA	2	2	4	4	*	4	4
Coconut macaroon Nabisco	2	190	2	10	23	NA	107	NA	*	2	2	*	*	4	4

Cookies (approx. 1 oz), cont'd.

Food	Serving	Calories	Protein g	Fat g	Carbo g	Fiber g	Sodium mg	Potassium mg	Vit A % rda	Vit B1 % rda (thiamin)	Vit B2 % rda (riboflavin)	Vit B3 % rda (niacin)	Vit C % rda	Calcium % rda	Iron % rda
Devil's food cakes Nabisco	2	140 ○	2 ○	1 ●	31 ○	NA	73 ●	NA	* ○	6 ○	4 ○	2 ○	* ○	* ○	4 ○
Fig Newtons	2	120 ○	1 ●	2 ●	22 ○	NA	125 ◐	NA	* ○	2 ○	2 ○	2 ○	2 ○	2 ○	4 ○
Fig Wheats Nabisco	2	120 ○	2 ●	2 ●	23 ○	NA	80 ●	* ○	2 ○	2 ○	2 ○	* ○	4 ○	4 ○	4 ○
Ginger man Pepperidge Farm	3	100 ○	1 ○	4 ●	15 ○	NA	75 ●	A	NA	NA	NA	NA	NA	NA	NA
Ginger snaps Nabisco	4	120 ○	2 ○	3 ●	22 ○	NA	75 ●	* ○	2 ○	2 ○	4 ○	4 ○	2 ○	2 ○	8 ○
Lemon crunch, small Pepperidge Farm	3	170 ○	1 ○	10 ○	19 ○	NA	75 ●	* ○	NA	4 ○	4 ○	* ○	NA	NA	NA
Lido	2	190 ○	1 ○	11 ○	21 ○	NA	85 ●	NA	NA	NA	NA	NA	NA	NA	NA
Lorna Doone	4	160 ○	2 ○	8 ○	20 ○	NA	183 ○	* ○	* ○	6 ○	6 ○	4 ○	* ○	* ○	4 ○
Macaroons	2	180 ○	2 ○	9 ○	25 ○	NA	14 ●	176 ○	0 ○	1 ○	4 ○	0 ○	1 ○	2 ○	2 ○
Mallomars	2	120 ○	1 ●	5 ○	17 ○	NA	50 ●	* ○	* ○	2 ○	2 ○	* ○	* ○	* ○	2 ○
Marshmallow Puff Nabisco	2	170 ○	1 ●	6 ○	28 ○	NA	80 ●	* ○	* ○	2 ○	4 ○	* ○	2 ○	2 ○	2 ○

Cookies (approx. 1 oz), cont'd.

Food	Serving	Calories	Protein g	Fat g	Carbo g	Fiber g	Sodium mg	Potassium mg	Vit A %rda	Vit B1 %rda (thiamin)	Vit B2 %rda (riboflavin)	Vit B3 %rda (niacin)	Vit C %rda	Calcium %rda	Iron %rda
Milano	3	180	1 ○	10 ○	21 ○	NA	80 ●	NA	NA	NA	NA	NA	NA	NA	NA
Mint Milano	2	153	0 ○	9 ○	17 ○	NA	70 ●	NA	NA	NA	NA	NA	NA	NA	NA
Mystic Mint	2	180	1 ○	9 ○	22 ○	NA	127 ●	NA	* ○	2 ○	2 ○	2 ○	* ○	4 ○	4 ○
Nassau	2	170	2 ○	10 ○	18 ○	NA	90 ●	NA	NA	NA	NA	NA	NA	NA	NA
Nilla wafers	7	130	1 ○	4 ●	21 ○	NA	95 ●	NA	* ○	4 ○	4 ○	4 ○	* ○	2 ○	2 ○
Oatmeal	2	118	2 ○	4 ●	19 ○	NA	111 ●	96 ○	0 ○	5 ○	3 ○	3 ○	* ○	1 ○	4 ○
Oatmeal raisin, slice 'n bake Pillsbury	3	160	2 ○	7 ○	22 ○	NA	75 ●	NA	0 ○	6 ○	4 ○	2 ○	0 ○	0 ○	4 ○
Oreo	3	150	2 ○	7 ●	22 ○	NA	210 ●	NA	* ○	* ○	2 ○	2 ○	* ○	4 ○	4 ○
Oreo Double Stuf	2	140	1 ○	7 ●	18 ○	NA	165 ●	NA	* ○	* ○	2 ○	2 ○	* ○	* ○	2 ○
Orleans	6	180	0 ○	12 ○	22 ○	NA	60 ●	NA	NA	NA	NA	NA	NA	NA	NA

Cookies (approx. 1 oz), cont'd.

Food	Serving	Calories	Protein g	Fat g	Carbo g	Fiber g	Sodium mg	Potassium mg	Vit A %rda	Vit B1 %rda (thiamin)	Vit B2 %rda (riboflavin)	Vit B3 %rda (niacin)	Vit C %rda	Calcium %rda	Iron %rda
Peanut butter chip Pepperidge Farm	3	160	2	9	19	NA	135	NA	NA	NA	NA	NA	NA	NA	NA
Peanut butter, slice 'n bake Pillsbury	3	170	3	9	19	NA	220	0	2	2	8	0	0	0	0
Pecan shortbread Nabisco	2	160	2	10	17	NA	85	*	6	4	4	*	*	2	2
Pinwheels, chocolate	1	140	1	6	21	NA	NA	*	2	2	*	*	*	2	2
Pirouettes Pepperidge Farm	3	110	0	7	13	NA	55	NA	NA	NA	NA	NA	NA	NA	NA
Raisin fruit biscuit, Nabisco	2	120	1	2	24	NA	NA	*	6	2	2	2	*	4	4
Sandwich	3	150	2	7	21	NA	144	11	3	4	3	0	0	1	3
Sandwich, fudge fudge Nabisco	3	160	2	7	23	NA	NA	*	2	4	2	*	*	4	4
Sandwich, marshmallow Nabisco	4	120	1	3	23	NA	97	*	2	4	2	*	*	2	2

Cookies (approx. 1 oz), cont'd.

Food	Serving	Calories	Protein g	Fat g	Carbo g	Fiber g	Sodium mg	Potassium mg	Vit A %rda	Vit B1 %rda (thiamin)	Vit B2 %rda (riboflavin)	Vit B3 %rda (niacin)	Vit C %rda	Calcium %rda	Iron %rda
Spiced wafers Nabisco	4	130	2	3	24	NA	228	NA	*	2	4	4	*	*	4
St Moritz	3	170	1	10	20	NA	70	NA	NA	NA	NA	NA	NA	NA	NA
Striped shortbread Nabisco	3	150	1	7	19	NA	80	NA	*	2	4	4	*	*	2
Sugar, slice 'n bake, Pillsbury	3	180	1	9	23	NA	210	0	0	6	0	2	0	2	2
Sugar, small Pepperidge Farm	2	150	1	8	20	NA	115	NA	NA	NA	NA	NA	NA	NA	NA
Tahiti	2	170	1	11	17	NA	50	NA	NA	NA	NA	NA	NA	NA	NA

Frostings

Food	Serving	Calories	Protein g	Fat g	Carbo g	Fiber g	Sodium mg	Potassium mg	Vit A %rda	Vit B1 %rda (thiamin)	Vit B2 %rda (riboflavin)	Vit B3 %rda (niacin)	Vit C %rda	Calcium %rda	Iron %rda
Creamy Deluxe, chocolate	1/12 cn	170	0	8	25	0	95	2	*	*	*	*	*	*	*
Creamy Deluxe, cream cheese	1/12 cn	170	0	7	27	0	100	0	*	*	*	*	*	*	*
Creamy Deluxe, orange	1/12 cn	170	0	6	28	0	95	0	*	*	*	*	*	*	*

Frostings, cont'd.

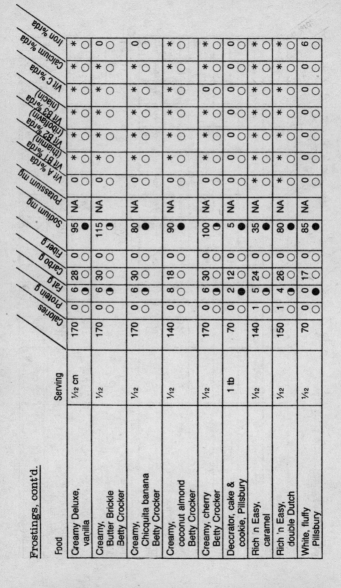

Food	Serving	Calories	Protein g	Fat g	Carbo g	Fiber g	Sodium mg	Potassium mg	Vit A %rda	Vit B1 %rda (thiamin)	Vit B2 %rda (riboflavin)	Vit B3 %rda (niacin)	Vit C %rda	Calcium %rda	Iron %rda
Creamy Deluxe, vanilla	1/12 cn	170	0 ○	6 ●	28 ○	0 ○	95 ●	NA	0 ○	* ○	* ○	* ○	* ○	* ○	* ○
Creamy, Butter Brickle Betty Crocker	1/12	170	0 ○	6 ●	30 ○	0 ○	115 ●	NA	0 ○	* ○	* ○	* ○	* ○	0 ○	0 ○
Creamy, Chicquita banana Betty Crocker	1/12	170	0 ○	6 ●	30 ○	0 ○	80 ●	NA	0 ○	* ○	* ○	* ○	* ○	0 ○	0 ○
Creamy, coconut almond Betty Crocker	1/12	140	0 ○	8 ○	18 ○	0 ○	90 ●	NA	0 ○	* ○	* ○	* ○	* ○	* ○	* ○
Creamy, cherry Betty Crocker	1/12	170	0 ○	6 ●	30 ○	0 ○	100 ●	NA	0 ○	* ○	* ○	* ○	* ○	* ○	* ○
Deccrator, cake & cookie, Pillsbury	1 tb	70	0 ○	2 ●	12 ○	0 ○	5 ●	NA	0 ○	0 ○	0 ○	0 ○	0 ○	0 ○	0 ○
Rich n Easy, caramel	1/12	140	1 ○	5 ●	24 ○	0 ○	35 ●	NA	* ○	* ○	* ○	* ○	* ○	* ○	* ○
Rich 'n Easy, double Dutch	1/12	150	1 ○	4 ●	26 ○	0 ○	80 ●	NA	* ○	* ○	* ○	* ○	* ○	* ○	* ○
White, fluffy Pillsbury	1/12	70	0 ●	0 ○	17 ○	0 ○	85 ●	NA	0 ○	0 ○	0 ○	0 ○	0 ○	0 ○	6 ○

Frozen Desserts

Food	Serving	Calories	Protein g	Fat g	Carbo g	Fiber g	Sodium mg	Potassium mg	Vit A %rda	Vit B1 %rda (thiamin)	Vit B2 %rda (riboflavin)	Vit B3 %rda (niacin)	Vit C %rda	Calcium %rda	Iron %rda
Bullwinkle pudding stix	1	120	2	5	20	0	NA	NA	*	*	2	*	*	15	2
Chocolate eclair Good Humor	1	220	1	13	25	0	NA	NA	*	*	2	*	2	2	*
Comet cone	1	20	0	0	4	0	NA	NA	*	*	*	*	*	*	*
Comet sugar cone	1	40	1	0	9	0	NA	NA	*	2	2	2	*	*	2
Creamsicle	1	78	1	3	13	0	14	41	2	NA	3	NA	3	3	*
Fudgsicle	1	104	3	0	24	0	34	111	3	3	15	1	11	11	2
Fudgsicle, banana	1	102	3	0	24	0	29	112	2	2	12	1	11	11	1
Ice cream bar, chocolate-coated Good Humor	1	170	2	13	12	0	NA	NA	*	*	6	*	6	6	*
Ice cream sandwich Good Humor	1	200	6	6	34	0	NA	NA	*	*	6	*	6	6	*
Ice cream, regular	1 c	270	5	14	32	0	106	257	3	3	19	2	18	18	1

Frozen Desserts, cont'd.

Food	Serving	Calories	Protein g	Fat g	Carbo g	Fiber g	Sodium mg	Potassium mg	Vit A % rda	Vit B1 % rda (thiamin)	Vit B2 % rda (riboflavin)	Vit B3 % rda (niacin)	Vit C % rda	Calcium % rda	Iron % rda
Ice cream, rich	1 c	350	4	24	32	0	49	221	18	3	16	1	2	15	1
Ice milk	1 c	185	5	6	29	0	105	265	4	5	21	1	2	18	1
Ice milk, soft-serve	1 c	225	8	5	38	0	163	412	4	8	32	1	2	27	2
Lite fruit stix Good Humor	1	35	0	0	8	0	NA	NA	*	*	*	*	*	*	*
Popsicle, fruit	1	70	0	0	17	0	9	1	0	0	0	0	0	0	0
Sandwich, chocolate chip cookie Good Humor	1	480	7	22	64	NA	NA	NA	10	4	10	*	*	8	6
Sherbet	1 c	270	2	4	59	0	89	198	4	2	5	7	7	10	2
Strawberry shortcake Good Humor	1	200	1	13	21	NA	NA	NA	*	2	2	*	*	2	*
Toasted almond bar Good Humor	1	220	2	14	21	NA	NA	NA	*	6	6	*	*	6	*

Frozen Desserts, cont'd.

Food	Serving	Calories	Protein g	Fat g	Carbo g	Fiber g	Sodium mg	Potassium mg	Vit A %rda	Vit B1 %rda (thiamin)	Vit B2 %rda (riboflavin)	Vit B3 %rda (niacin)	Vit C %rda	Calcium %rda	Iron %rda
Whammy	1	100	1 ○	7 ●	9 ○	NA	NA	NA	* ○	* ○	2 ○	* ○	2 ○	* ○	* ○
Whammy chip crunch	1	110	1 ○	7 ●	10 ○	NA	NA	NA	* ○	* ○	2 ○	* ○	2 ○	* ○	* ○

Gelatin

Food	Serving	Calories	Protein g	Fat g	Carbo g	Fiber g	Sodium mg	Potassium mg	Vit A %rda	Vit B1 %rda (thiamin)	Vit B2 %rda (riboflavin)	Vit B3 %rda (niacin)	Vit C %rda	Calcium %rda	Iron %rda
All flavors Royal	½ c	80	2 ○	0 ●	19 ○	0	90 ●	1 ○	* ○	* ○	* ○	* ○	15 ○	* ○	* ○
D-zerta, all flavors	½ c	8	2 ○	0 ●	0 ○	0	9 ●	50 ○	* ○	* ○	* ○	* ○	* ○	* ○	* ○
Sweet As You Please	½ c	6	1 ○	0 ●	0 ○	0	90 ●	1 ○	* ○	* ○	* ○	* ○	* ○	* ○	* ○

Jams and Jellies

Food	Serving	Calories	Protein g	Fat g	Carbo g	Fiber g	Sodium mg	Potassium mg	Vit A %rda	Vit B1 %rda (thiamin)	Vit B2 %rda (riboflavin)	Vit B3 %rda (niacin)	Vit C %rda	Calcium %rda	Iron %rda
Jam	1 tb	55	0 ○	0 ●	14 ○	0	2 ●	18 ○	* ○	* ○	1 ○	* ○	0 ○	1 ○	* ○
Jelly	1 tb	50	0 ○	0 ●	13 ○	0	3 ●	14 ○	* ○	* ○	1 ○	2 ○	0 ○	2 ○	* ○

Pastry

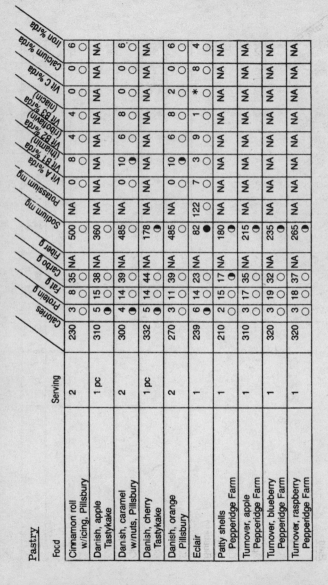

Food	Serving	Calories	Protein g	Fat g	Carbo g	Fiber g	Sodium mg	Potassium mg	Vit A %rda	Vit B1 %rda (thiamin)	Vit B2 %rda (riboflavin)	Vit B3 %rda (niacin)	Vit C %rda	Calcium %rda	Iron %rda
Cinnamon roll w/icing, Pillsbury	2	230	3	8	35	NA	500	NA	0	4	4	0	0	6	6
Danish, apple Tastykake	1 pc	310	5	15	38	NA	360	NA	NA	NA	NA	NA	NA	NA	NA
Danish, caramel w/nuts, Pillsbury	2	300	4	14	39	NA	485	NA	10	6	8	0	0	6	6
Danish, cherry Tastykake	1 pc	332	5	14	44	NA	178	NA	NA	NA	NA	NA	NA	NA	NA
Danish, orange Pillsbury	2	270	3	11	39	NA	485	NA	10	6	8	2	0	6	6
Eclair	1	239	6	23	NA	NA	82	122	3	9	1	*	8	4	4
Patty shells Pepperidge Farm	1	210	2	15	17	NA	180	NA	NA	NA	NA	NA	NA	NA	NA
Turnover, apple Pepperidge Farm	1	310	3	17	35	NA	215	NA	NA	NA	NA	NA	NA	NA	NA
Turnover, blueberry Pepperidge Farm	1	320	3	19	32	NA	235	NA	NA	NA	NA	NA	NA	NA	NA
Turnover, raspberry Pepperidge Farm	1	320	3	18	37	NA	265	NA	NA	NA	NA	NA	NA	NA	NA

Pies

Food	Serving	Calories	Protein g	Fat g	Carbo g	Fiber g	Sodium mg	Potassium mg	Vit A %rda	Vit B1 %rda (thiamin)	Vit B2 %rda (riboflavin)	Vit B3 %rda (niacin)	Vit C %rda	Calcium %rda	Iron %rda
Apple, 9-in	1/6	403	4	18	60	NA	461	126	1	12	8	8	4	1	6
Apple, Tastykake	1 pc	362	4	14	52	NA	458	NA	NA	NA	NA	NA	NA	NA	NA
Banana cream Pet-Ritz	1/6	170	2	9	22	NA		NA	NA	4	2	3	NA	2	5
Blueberry Tastykake	1 pc	376	3	11	62	NA	406	NA	NA	NA	NA	NA	NA	NA	NA
Blueberry, 9-in	1/6	379	4	18	55	NA	361	103	1	12	8	8	8	2	9
Cherry, 9-in	1/6	408	5	18	61	NA	374	166	14	12	8	8	NA	2	6
Chocolate cream Pet-Ritz	1/6	190	1	8	27	NA		NA	NA	5	2	3	NA	2	5
Cobbler, apple 11 oz Pet-Ritz	1/2	370	1	12	64	NA	NA	NA	*	*	3	*	3	*	3
Cobbler, blackberry 11 oz Pet-Ritz	1/2	325	3	13	50	NA	NA	NA	*	*	5	4	5	*	6
Cobbler, peach, 11 oz, Pet-Ritz	1/2	365	3	13	60	NA	NA	NA	8	5	3	3	14	*	*

Pies, cont'd.

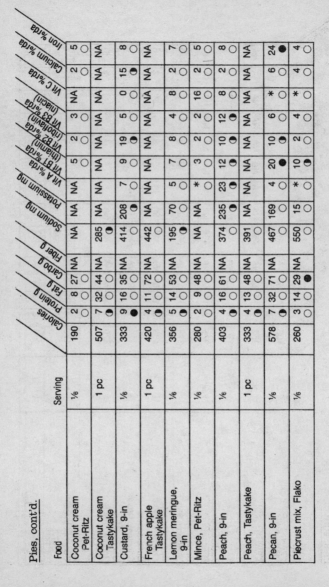

Food	Serving	Calories	Protein g	Fat g	Carbo g	Fiber g	Sodium mg	Potassium mg	Vit A %rda	Vit B1 %rda (thiamin)	Vit B2 %rda (riboflavin)	Vit B3 %rda (niacin)	Vit C %rda	Calcium %rda	Iron %rda
Coconut cream Pet-Ritz	1/6	190	2○	8○	27○	NA	NA	NA	5○	2○	3○	NA	2○	2○	5○
Coconut cream Tastykake	1 pc	507	7●	32○	44	NA	285●	NA	NA	NA	NA	NA	NA	NA	NA
Custard, 9-in	1/6	333	9●	16○	35○	NA	414○	208●	7○	9○	19●	5○	0○	15●	8○
French apple Tastykake	1 pc	420	4●	11○	72○	NA	442○	NA	NA	NA	NA	NA	NA	NA	NA
Lemon meringue, 9-in	1/6	356	5●	14○	53○	NA	195●	70○	7○	7○	8○	8○	8○	2○	7○
Mince, Pet-Ritz	1/6	280	2○	9○	48○	NA	NA	*○	3○	3○	2○	16○	16○	2○	5○
Peach, 9-in	1/6	403	4●	16○	61○	NA	374○	235●	12●	12●	10●	8○	8○	2○	8○
Peach, Tastykake	1 pc	333	4●	13○	48○	NA	391○	NA	NA	NA	NA	NA	NA	NA	NA
Pecan, 9-in	1/6	578	7●	32○	71○	NA	467○	169○	20●	10○	10○	*○	6○	6○	24●
Piecrust mix, Flako	1/6	260	3○	14○	29●	NA	550○	15○	10○	2○	4○	*○	4○	4○	4○

Pies, cont'd.

Food	Serving	Calories	Protein g	Fat g	Carbo g	Fiber g	Sodium mg	Potassium mg	Vit A %rda	Vit B1 %rda (thiamin)	Vit B2 %rda (riboflavin)	Vit B3 %rda (niacin)	Vit C %rda	Calcium %rda	Iron %rda
Pumpkin custard Pet-Ritz	⅙	250 ○	4 ●	9 ○	39 ○	NA	NA	NA	28 ●	3 ○	* ○	* ○	2 ○	6 ○	2 ○
Pumpkin, 9-in	⅙	321 ●	18 ○	6 ●	37 ○	NA	361 ○	243 ●	75 ●	9 ○	12 ●	6 ○	* ○	8 ○	7 ○

Puddings and Custards

Food	Serving	Calories	Protein g	Fat g	Carbo g	Fiber g	Sodium mg	Potassium mg	Vit A %rda	Vit B1 %rda (thiamin)	Vit B2 %rda (riboflavin)	Vit B3 %rda (niacin)	Vit C %rda	Calcium %rda	Iron %rda
Banana cream, instant, Jell-O	½ c	170 ●	4 ●	4 ●	30 ○	0 ○	185 ○	2 ○	2 ○	10 ●	* ○	* ○	15 ●	* ○	2 ○
Butter pecan, instant, Jell-O	½ c	170 ●	4 ●	5 ●	29 ○	0 ○	195 ○	2 ○	4 ○	10 ●	* ○	* ○	15 ●	* ○	2 ○
Butterscotch instant, Royal	½ c	180 ●	4 ●	5 ●	29 ○	0 ○	145 ○	4 ○	2 ○	15 ●	* ○	2 ○	15 ●	2 ○	* ○
Chocolate fudge, instant, Jell-O	½ c	180 ●	5 ●	5 ●	32 ○	0 ○	210 ○	2 ○	4 ○	15 ●	* ○	* ○	15 ●	2 ○	4 ○
Chocolate instant Royal	½ c	190 ●	4 ●	4 ●	35 ○	0 ○	235 ●	4 ○	* ○	20 ●	* ○	2 ○	15 ●	4 ○	4 ○
Coconut instant Royal	½ c	170 ●	4 ●	4 ●	30 ○	0 ○	185 ●	4 ○	2 ○	15 ●	* ○	2 ○	15 ●	2 ○	2 ○
Custard & flan Royal	½ c	150 ●	4 ●	5 ●	22 ○	0 ○	130 ●	4 ○	2 ○	20 ●	* ○	2 ○	15 ●	2 ○	* ○

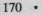

Puddings and Custards, cont'd.

Food	Serving	Calories	Protein g	Fat g	Carbo g	Fiber g	Sodium mg	Potassium mg	Vit A %rda	VR B1 %rda (thiamin)	VR B2 %rda (riboflavin)	VR B3 %rda (niacin)	Vit C %rda	Calcium %rda	Iron %rda
Custard, baked	½ c	153	7	8	15	0	104	194	9	4	15	1	1	15	3
D-zerta, butterscotch	½ c	70	4	0	12	0	145	235	4	4	10	*	2	15	*
D-zerta, chocolate	½ c	70	5	0	11	0	80	225	4	2	10	*	2	15	*
Egg custard, Golden Jell-O	½ c	160	5	5	23	0	220	255	4	6	15	*	*	20	2
French vanilla, noninstant, Jell-O	½ c	170	4	4	30	0	200	185	2	2	10	*	*	15	*
Milk chocolate, noninstant, Jell-O	½ c	170	5	4	29	0	180	210	2	4	15	*	*	15	*
Pineapple cream, instant, Jell-O	½ c	170	4	4	30	0	335	185	2	2	10	2	*	15	*
Rice, Jell-O	½ c	170	5	4	30	0	155	185	2	6	10	*	*	15	*
Snack Pack, chocolate	1	180	3	7	28	0	NA	NA	*	*	6	*	*	8	6
Snack Pack, banana	1	180	2	9	24	0	NA	NA	*	*	6	*	*	8	*
Snack Pack, rice	1	190	3	9	27	0	NA	NA	*	2	6	*	*	10	*

Puddings and Custards, cont'd.

Food	Serving	Calories	Protein g	Fat g	Carbo g	Fiber g	Sodium mg	Potassium mg	Vit A %rda	Vit B1 %rda (thiamin)	Vit B2 %rda (riboflavin)	Vit B3 %rda (niacin)	Vit C %rda	Calcium %rda	Iron %rda
Snack Pack, tapioca	1	140	3	4	23	0	NA	NA	*	*	8	*	10	*	*
Snack Pack, vanilla	1	180	2	7	29	0	NA	NA	*	*	6	*	8	*	*
Vanilla instant Royal	½ c	180	4	5	29	0	245	145	4	2	15	2	15	15	*
Vanilla tapioca Royal	½ c	160	4	4	27	0	225	150	4	2	10	2	15	15	*

Snacks

Food	Serving	Calories	Protein g	Fat g	Carbo g	Fiber g	Sodium mg	Potassium mg	Vit A %rda	Vit B1 %rda (thiamin)	Vit B2 %rda (riboflavin)	Vit B3 %rda (niacin)	Vit C %rda	Calcium %rda	Iron %rda
Baken-ets	1 oz	150	17	9	1	NA	570	NA	*	*	2	*	*	*	*
Breakfast bar, chocolate chip Carnation	1	200	6	11	21	NA	165	103	20	25	25	45	2	25	25
Breakfast bar, chocolate crunch Carnation	1	190	6	10	18	NA	130	107	20	25	25	45	2	25	25

Snacks, cont'd.

Food	Serving	Calories	Protein g	Fat g	Carbo g	Fiber g	Sodium mg	Potassium mg	Vit A %rda	Vit B1 %rda (thiamin)	Vit B2 %rda (riboflavin)	Vit B3 %rda (niacin)	Vit C %rda	Calcium %rda	Iron %rda
Breakfast bar, peanut butter Carnation	1	180	6●	9○	20○	NA	155●	68○	35●	20●	25●	45●	2○	2○	25●
Bugles	1 oz	150	2○	8●	18●	NA	335○	NA	*○	2○	4○	*○	*○	4○	4○
Carob raisins Flavor Tree	1 oz	130	1○	5●	20○	NA	NA	NA	2○	*○	2○	*○	2○	2○	2○
Cheddar chips Flavor Tree	1 oz	160	3○	11○	12○	NA	NA	NA	2○	*○	2○	*○	4○	4○	4○
Cheetos	1 oz	160	2○	10○	15○	NA	260●	NA	4○	*○	4○	*○	*○	*○	4○
Chewing gum	1 pc	5	0●	0○	2○	0○	NA	NA	0○	0○	0○	0○	NA	NA	NA
Corn Dogs Oscar Mayer	1	330	10●	20○	27●	NA	1252○	164○	18●	9○	16●	5○	3○	10●	10●
Corn Korkers	19	160	2○	10●	16●	NA	NA	NA	*○	*○	*○	*○	2○	2○	2○
Crunch mix, sesame coconut Flavor Tree	1 oz	130	1○	5●	20●	NA	NA	*○	2○	2○	2○	*○	4○	2○	2○

Snacks, cont'd.

Food	Serving	Calories	Protein g	Fat g	Carbo g	Fiber g	Sodium mg	Potassium mg	Vit A %rda	Vit B1 %rda (thiamin)	Vit B2 %rda (riboflavin)	Vit B3 %rda (niacin)	Vit C %rda	Calcium %rda	Iron %rda
Crunch mix, sesame honey Flavor Tree	1 oz	140	2	7	18	NA	NA	NA	*	4	*	2	*	6	2
Dip, French onion Kraft	2 tb	60	1	4	3	NA	240	6	*	*	*	*	*	*	*
Dip, avocado Kraft	2 tb	50	1	4	3	NA	215	*	*	*	*	*	*	*	*
Doo Dads	57	140	3	7	17	NA	380	*	6	4	8	*	2	4	4
Doritos	1 oz	140	2	7	19	NA	NA	*	*	*	*	*	2	2	2
Doritos, taco-flavored	1 oz	140	2	7	18	NA	185	2	4	2	*	2	2	2	2
Food sticks, caramel Pillsbury	4	180	4	6	27	NA	165	6	6	3	6	6	6	6	6
Food sticks, chocolate Pillsbury	4	180	4	6	27	NA	115	6	6	6	6	6	6	6	6
Food sticks, chocolate mint Pillsbury	4	180	4	6	27	NA	95	6	6	6	6	6	6	6	6

Snacks, cont'd.

Food	Serving	Calories	Protein g	Fat g	Carbo g	Fiber g	Sodium mg	Potassium mg	Vit A %rda	Vit B1 %rda (thiamin)	Vit B2 %rda (riboflavin)	Vit B3 %rda (niacin)	Vit C %rda	Calcium %rda	Iron %rda
Food sticks, orange Pillsbury	4	180	4	6	27	NA	135	NA	6	6	6	6	6	6	6
French onion crisp Flavor Tree	1 oz	150	3	9	13	NA	NA	NA	*	2	*	2	*	4	4
Fritos corn chips	1 oz	150	2	9	16	NA	180	NA	*	*	*	*	*	4	*
Fruit Roll-ups, all flavors	1	50	0	1	12	NA	NA	NA	*	*	*	*	*	*	*
Goldfish, cheddar cheese Pepperidge Farm	45	140	3	6	18	NA	175	NA	NA	NA	NA	NA	NA	NA	NA
Granola & fruit bar apple Nature Valley	1	140	2	4	25	NA	150	NA	*	2	*	*	*	*	4
Granola & fruit bar date, Nature Valley	1	140	2	4	25	NA	130	NA	*	2	*	*	*	2	4
Granola & fruit bar raspberry Nature Valley	1	150	2	5	25	NA	160	NA	*	2	*	*	2	*	2
Granola bar, cinnamon Nature Valley	1	110	2	4	16	NA	65	NA	*	4	*	*	*	*	4

Snacks, cont'd.

Food	Serving	Calories	Protein g	Fat g	Carbo g	Fiber g	Sodium mg	Potassium mg	Vit A %rda	Vit B1 %rda (thiamin)	Vit B2 %rda (riboflavin)	Vit B3 %rda (niacin)	Vit C %rda	Calcium % rda	Iron % rda
Granola bar, coconut Nature Valley	1	120	2 ○	6 ●	15 ○	NA	65 ●	NA	4 ○	* ○	* ○	* ○	* ○	4 ○	4 ○
Granola bar, oats 'n honey Nature Valley	1	110	2 ○	4 ●	16 ○	NA	65 ●	NA	4 ○	* ○	* ○	* ○	* ○	4 ○	4 ○
Granola bar, almond Nature Valley	1	110	2 ○	4 ●	16 ○	NA	80 ●	NA	4 ○	2 ○	* ○	* ○	* ○	4 ○	4 ○
Granola clusters, almond Nature Valley	1	140	3 ○	3 ●	27 ○	NA	140 ●	NA	4 ○	2 ○	* ○	* ○	2 ○	4 ○	4 ○
Granola clusters, caramel Nature Valley	1	150	3 ○	3 ●	28 ○	NA	15 ●	NA	4 ○	2 ○	* ○	* ○	2 ○	2 ○	2 ○
Granola clusters, raisin Nature Valley	1	150	3 ○	3 ●	28 ○	NA	110 ●	NA	4 ○	* ○	* ○	* ○	2 ○	2 ○	2 ○
Light & Crunchy granola snack, cinnamon	1 pk	140	2 ○	6 ●	19 ○	NA	175 ●	NA	2 ○	* ○	* ○	* ○	2 ○	2 ○	2 ○
Light & Crunchy granola snack, oats 'n honey	1 pk	140	2 ○	7 ●	18 ○	NA	170 ●	NA	2 ○	* ○	* ○	* ○	2 ○	2 ○	2 ○

Snacks, cont'd.

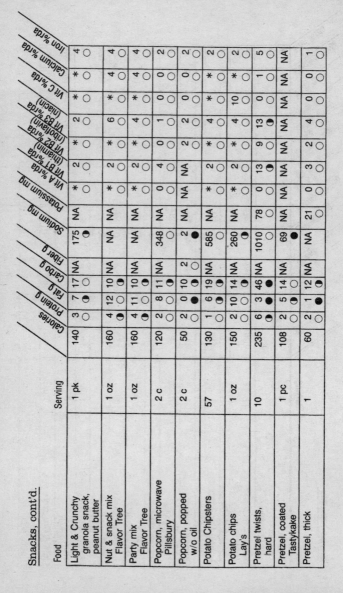

Food	Serving	Calories	Protein g	Fat g	Carbo g	Fiber g	Sodium mg	Potassium mg	Vit A %rda	Vit B1 %rda (thiamin)	Vit B2 %rda (riboflavin)	Vit B3 %rda (niacin)	Vit C %rda	Calcium %rda	Iron %rda
Light & Crunchy granola snack, peanut butter	1 pk	140	3	7	17	NA	175	*	*	2	*	2	*	4	4
Nut & snack mix Flavor Tree	1 oz	160	4	12	10	NA	NA	*	2	2	6	*	4	4	4
Party mix Flavor Tree	1 oz	160	4	11	10	NA	NA	*	2	2	4	*	4	4	4
Popcorn, microwave Pillsbury	2 c	120	2	8	11	NA	348	0	4	4	1	0	0	2	2
Popcorn, popped w/o oil	2 c	50	2	0	10	2	2	NA	NA	2	2	0	0	2	2
Potato Chipsters	57	130	1	6	19	NA	585	*	*	*	*	*	*	2	2
Potato chips Lay's	1 oz	150	2	10	14	NA	260	*	2	*	4	10	*	2	2
Pretzel twists, hard	10	235	6	3	46	NA	1010	0	13	13	9	0	1	5	5
Pretzel, coated Tastykake	1 pc	108	5	14	NA	NA	69	NA	NA	NA	2	NA	NA	NA	NA
Pretzel, thick	1	60	1	12	NA	NA	21	0	3	2	2	0	0	1	1

Snacks, cont'd.

Food	Serving	Calories	Protein g	Fat g	Carbo g	Fiber g	Sodium mg	Potassium mg	Vit A %rda	Vit B1 %rda (thiamin)	Vit B2 %rda (riboflavin)	Vit B3 %rda (niacin)	Vit C %rda	Calcium %rda	Iron %rda
Pretzels, Dutch style Rokeach	1 oz	110	3 ○	0 ●	24 ●	NA	NA	NA	* ○	* ○	* ○	* ○	* ○	* ○	* ○
Pretzels, unsalted Rokeach	1 oz	110	2 ○	0 ●	20 ●	NA	30 ●	NA	* ○	* ○	* ○	* ○	* ○	* ○	* ○
Sesame bran stick Flavor Tree	1 oz	160	3 ○	11 ○	11 ●	NA	NA	NA	* ○	* ○	2 ○	* ○	4 ○	4 ○	4 ○
Sesame buds Flavor Tree	1 oz	170	3 ○	13 ○	10 ●	NA	NA	NA	* ○	2 ○	2 ○	* ○	6 ○	6 ○	6 ○
Sesame buds w/garlic Flavor Tree	1 oz	160	3 ○	11 ○	12 ●	NA	NA	NA	* ○	2 ○	2 ○	* ○	4 ○	4 ○	4 ○
Snack bar, apple nut Pepperidge Farm	1	170	1 ○	5 ●	33 ○	NA	90 ●	NA	NA	NA	NA	NA	NA	NA	NA
Snack bar, blueberry Pepperidge Farm	1	170	1 ○	3 ●	36 ○	NA	90 ●	NA	NA	NA	NA	NA	NA	NA	NA
Snack bar, brownie nut Pepperidge Farm	1	190	2 ○	7 ●	30 ○	NA	100 ●	NA	NA	NA	NA	NA	NA	NA	NA

Snacks, cont'd.

Food	Serving	Calories	Protein g	Fat g	Carbo g	Fiber g	Sodium mg	Potassium mg	Vit A %rda	Vit B1 %rda (thiamin)	Vit B2 %rda (riboflavin)	Vit B3 %rda (niacin)	Vit C %rda	Calcium %rda	Iron %rda
Snack bar, date nut Pepperidge Farm	1	190	2○	7●	30○	NA	90●	NA	NA	NA	NA	NA	NA	NA	NA
Snack mix, sunflower sesame Flavor Tree	1 oz	170	5●	13●	8○	NA	NA	*○	10●	4○	2○	*○	4○	10●	NA
Snack sticks, parmesan pretzel Pepperidge Farm	8	120	2○	3●	21●	NA	195●	NA	NA	NA	NA	NA	NA	NA	NA
Snack sticks, pumpernickel Pepperidge Farm	8	130	2○	5●	20●	NA	380○	NA	NA	NA	NA	NA	NA	NA	NA
Snack sticks, salted Pepperidge Farm	8	130	2○	5●	20●	NA	320●	NA	NA	NA	NA	NA	NA	NA	NA

Sugars

Food	Serving	Calories	Protein g	Fat g	Carbo g	Fiber g	Sodium mg	Potassium mg	Vit A %rda	Vit B1 %rda (thiamin)	Vit B2 %rda (riboflavin)	Vit B3 %rda (niacin)	Vit C %rda	Calcium %rda	Iron %rda
Brown packed	1 c	820	0○	0○	212○	0○	66●	757●	1○	4○	2○	0○	0○	19●	42●
Granulated	1 ts	15	0○	0●	4○	0○	0●	0○	0○	0○	0○	0○	0○	0○	*○

Sugars, cont'd.

Food	Serving	Calories	Protein g	Fat g	Carbo g	Fiber g	Sodium mg	Potassium mg	Vit A %rda	Vit B1 %rda (thiamin)	Vit B2 %rda (riboflavin)	Vit B3 %rda (niacin)	Vit C %rda	Calcium %rda	Iron %rda
Powdered	1 c	385	0	0	100	0	0	3	0	0	0	0	0	1	1
Sprinkle sweet	1/8 ts	2	0	0	0	0	1	NA	*	*	*	*	*	*	*
Sweet 10	1/8 ts	0	0	0	0	0	2	NA	*	*	*	*	*	*	*

Syrups

Food	Serving	Calories	Protein g	Fat g	Carbo g	Fiber g	Sodium mg	Potassium mg	Vit A %rda	Vit B1 %rda (thiamin)	Vit B2 %rda (riboflavin)	Vit B3 %rda (niacin)	Vit C %rda	Calcium %rda	Iron %rda
Chocolate	2 tb	90	1	1	24	0	20	106	*	0	2	0	1	3	3
Corn	1 tb	60	0	0	15	0	14	1	0	0	0	0	1	4	0
Fudge	2 tb	125	2	5	20	0	34	107	*	1	5	*	5	3	3
Honey	1 tb	65	0	0	17	0	1	11	0	0	1	*	0	1	1
Molasses, blackstrap	1 tb	45	0	0	11	0	18	585	1	2	2	NA	14	18	18
Molasses, light	1 tb	50	0	0	13	0	3	183	1	*	1	NA	3	5	5

Syrups, cont'd.

Food	Serving	Calories	Protein g	Fat g	Carbo g	Fiber g	Sodium mg	Potassium mg	Vit A %rda	Vit B1 %rda (thiamin)	Vit B2 %rda (riboflavin)	Vit B3 %rda (niacin)	Vit C %rda	Calcium %rda	Iron %rda
Pancake Aunt Jemima	2 tb	100	0	0	26	0	25	10	*	*	*	*	*	*	*
Pancake, Lite Aunt Jemima	2 tb	60	0	0	15	0	65	9	*	*	*	*	*	*	*
Pancake, substitute Tillie Lewis	2 tb	8	0	0	2	0	NA	NA	*	*	*	*	*	*	*
Topping, caramel Kraft	2 tb	100	2	0	24	0	90	NA	*	*	4	*	4	*	*
Topping, chocolate, lo-cal Tillie Lewis	2 tb	16	0	0	4	0	NA	NA	*	*	*	*	*	*	*
Topping, pineapple Kraft	2 tb	100	0	0	26	0	10	NA	*	*	*	*	*	*	*
Topping, strawberry Kraft	2 tb	90	0	0	22	0	10	NA	*	*	*	12	*	*	*
Topping, walnut Kraft	2 tb	180	2	10	20	0	10	NA	*	*	*	*	*	*	*

Odds & Ends
Condiments

Food	Serving	Calories	Protein g	Fat g	Carbo g	Fiber g	Sodium mg	Potassium mg	Vit A %rda	Vit B1 %rda (thiamin)	Vit B2 %rda (riboflavin)	Vit B3 %rda (niacin)	Vit C %rda	Calcium %rda	Iron %rda
Apple butter	1 tb	33	0	0	8	0	1	44	*	*	*	*	0	1	1
BacOs	1 tb	40	3	2	2	0	230	NA	45	0	*	*	*	2	2
Bitters, aromatic Angostura	1 ts	15	0	0	1	0	0	NA	0	0	0	0	*	*	*
Catsup	1 tb	15	0	0	4	0	156	54	1	1	1	3	*	*	1
Catsup, imitation Tillie Lewis	1 tb	8	0	0	2	0	9	NA	*	*	*	*	*	*	*
Chili-O	1/6 pk	25	1	0	5	0	630	*	*	*	2	*	*	*	*
Garlic clove	1	4	0	0	1	0	1	*	1	1	*	*	0	*	*
Horseradish sauce Kraft	1 tb	50	0	5	2	0	100	16	*	*	*	*	*	*	*
Horseradish Kraft	1 tb	4	0	0	1	0	50	NA	*	*	*	*	*	*	*
Marinade, meat French's	1/8 pk	10	0	0	2	0	540	NA	*	*	*	2	*	*	*
Mayonnaise	1 tb	100	0	11	0	0	72	5	*	*	1	NA	0	1	1

Condiments, cont'd.

Food	Serving	Calories	Protein g	Fat g	Carbo g	Fiber g	Sodium mg	Potassium mg	Vit A %rda	Vit B1 %rda (thiamin)	Vit B2 %rda (riboflavin)	Vit B3 %rda (niacin)	Vit C %rda	Calcium %rda	Iron %rda
Meat tenderizer French's	1 ts	2 ○	0 ○	0 ●	0 ○	0 ○	1760 ○	NA	* ○	* ○	* ○	* ○	* ○	* ○	* ○
Miracle Whip	1 tb	70 ○	0 ○	7 ●	2 ○	0 ○	85 ●	NA	* ○	* ○	* ○	* ○	* ○	* ○	* ○
Mustard, Bold 'n Spicy, French's	1 tb	16 ○	1 ○	1 ●	1 ○	NA	145 ●	NA	* ○	* ○	* ○	* ○	* ○	* ○	* ○
Mustard, Medford French's	1 tb	16 ○	1 ○	1 ●	1 ○	NA	240 ●	NA	* ○	* ○	* ○	* ○	* ○	* ○	* ○
Mustard, prepared	1 ts	5 ○	0 ○	0 ●	0 ○	0 ○	64 ●	7 ○	NA	NA	NA	NA	0 ○	1 ○	1 ○
Olive, green	3	15 ○	0 ○	2 ●	0 ○	0 ○	323 ●	7 ○	1 ○	NA	NA	NA	1 ○	1 ○	1 ○
Olive, mission	3	15 ○	0 ○	2 ●	0 ○	0 ○	65 ●	2 ○	0 ○	NA	* ○	NA	1 ○	1 ○	1 ○
Pepper, seasoned French's	1 ts	8 ○	0 ○	0 ●	1 ○	0 ○	5 ●	NA	* ○	* ○	* ○	* ○	* ○	* ○	* ○
Pickle	2 sl	10 ○	0 ○	0 ●	3 ○	0 ○	215 ●	NA	0 ○	* ○	* ○	2 ○	1 ○	2 ○	2 ○
Pickle, dill, medium	1	5 ○	0 ○	0 ●	1 ○	0 ○	928 ○	130 ○	1 ○	* ○	1 ○	7 ○	1 ○	4 ○	1 ○
Pickle, sweet	1	20 ○	0 ○	0 ●	5 ○	0 ○	NA	NA	0 ○	* ○	* ○	2 ○	0 ○	1 ○	0 ○

Condiments, cont'd.

Food	Serving	Calories	Protein g	Fat g	Carbo g	Fiber g	Sodium mg	Potassium mg	Vit A %rda	Vit B1 %rda (thiamin)	Vit B2 %rda (riboflavin)	Vit B3 %rda (niacin)	Vit C %rda	Calcium %rda	Iron %rda
Pimentos, 4-oz jar Dromedary	¼	10	0	0	2	NA	NA	10	*	*	*	*	15	*	8
Relish	1 tb	20	0	0	5	0	107	NA	NA	NA	NA	NA	NA	0	1
Salad dressing, Mayo-type, whipped	1 tb	65	0	6	2	0	88	1	*	*	*	*	NA	0	*
Salt	1 ts	0	0	0	0	0	2132	0	0	0	0	0	0	*	0
Salt, butter flavor French's	1 ts	8	1	0	0	0	1125	*	*	*	*	*	*	*	*
Salt, celery French's	1 ts	2	0	0	0	0	1505	NA	*	*	*	*	*	*	*
Salt, garlic French's	1 ts	4	0	0	1	0	2050	NA	*	*	*	*	*	*	*
Salt, garlic, parslied, French's	1 ts	6	0	0	1	0	1125	NA	*	*	*	*	*	*	*
Salt, hickory smoke French's	1 ts	2	0	0	0	0	1145	NA	*	*	*	*	*	*	*
Salt, onion French's	1 ts	6	0	0	1	0	1590	NA	*	*	*	*	*	*	*
Salt, seasoned French's	1 ts	2	0	0	1	0	1280	NA	*	*	*	*	*	*	*

Condiments, cont'd.

Food	Serving	Calories	Protein g	Fat g	Carbo g	Fiber g	Sodium mg	Potassium mg	Vit A %rda	Vit B1 %rda (thiamin)	Vit B2 %rda (riboflavin)	Vit B3 %rda (niacin)	Vit C %rda	Calcium %rda	Iron %rda
Seasoning, beef stew, French's	⅙ pk	25	0 ○	0 ●	5 ○	0 ○	765 ○	NA	* ○	* ○	2 ○	* ○	* ○	2 ○	2 ○
Seasoning, enchilada, French's	¼ pk	30	1 ○	1 ●	5 ○	0 ○	1130 ○	NA	* ○	* ○	2 ○	* ○	* ○	2 ○	2 ○
Seasoning, hamburger, French's	¼ pk	25	1 ○	0 ●	5 ○	0 ○	450 ○	NA	* ○	* ○	* ○	* ○	2 ○	* ○	* ○
Seasoning, sloppy Joe French's	⅛ pk	16	0 ○	0 ●	4 ○	0 ○	390 ○	NA	* ○	* ○	* ○	* ○	* ○	* ○	* ○
Seasoning, lemon & pepper, French's	1 ts	6	0 ○	0 ●	1 ○	0 ○	805 ○	NA	* ○	* ○	* ○	* ○	* ○	* ○	* ○
Seasoning, meatball French's	¼ pk	35	1 ○	0 ●	7 ○	0 ○	825 ○	NA	* ○	* ○	* ○	* ○	* ○	* ○	2 ○
Seasoning, meatloaf French's	⅛ pk	20	1 ○	0 ●	5 ○	0 ○	615 ○	NA	* ○	* ○	* ○	* ○	* ○	* ○	* ○
Seasoning, seafood French's	1 ts	2	0 ○	0 ●	0 ○	0 ○	1410 ○	NA	* ○	* ○	* ○	* ○	* ○	* ○	* ○
Seasoning, taco French's	⅙ pk	20	1 ○	0 ●	4 ○	0 ○	365 ○	NA	* ○	* ○	* ○	* ○	* ○	* ○	* ○
Soy sauce, La Choy	1 tb	8	1 ○	0 ●	1 ○	0 ○	975 ○	NA	NA	NA	NA	NA	NA	NA	NA

Condiments, cont'd.

Food	Serving	Calories	Protein g	Fat g	Carbo g	Fiber g	Sodium mg	Potassium mg	Vit A %rda	Vit B1 %rda (thiamin)	Vit B2 %rda (riboflavin)	Vit B3 %rda (niacin)	Vit C %rda	Calcium %rda	Iron %rda
Sugar, cinnamon French's	1 ts	16	0	0	4	0	0	NA	*	*	*	*	*	*	*
Tabasco sauce	1 ts	0	0	0	0	0	22	3	*	*	*	NA	NA	NA	NA
Tartar sauce	1 tb	75	0	8	1	0	99	11	*	*	1	*	0	1	1
Vegetable flakes, dehydrated French's	1 tb	12	0	0	3	NA	20	NA	*	*	*	*	*	*	*
Worcestershire sauce, French's	1 tb	10	0	0	2	0	165	NA	*	*	*	*	*	*	*

Fats and Oils

Food	Serving	Calories	Protein g	Fat g	Carbo g	Fiber g	Sodium mg	Potassium mg	Vit A %rda	Vit B1 %rda (thiamin)	Vit B2 %rda (riboflavin)	Vit B3 %rda (niacin)	Vit C %rda	Calcium %rda	Iron %rda
Butter	1 tb	100	0	12	0	0	116	4	9	*	*	0	0	*	*
Butter, whipped	1 tb	65	0	8	0	0	74	2	6	*	*	0	0	*	*
Corn oil	1 tb	120	0	14	0	0	0	NA	0	0	0	0	0	0	0

Fats and Oils, cont'd.

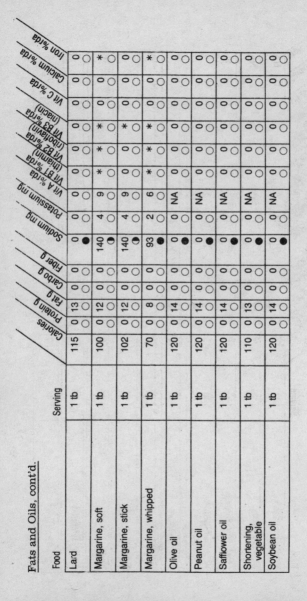

Food	Serving	Calories	Protein g	Fat g	Carbo g	Fiber g	Sodium mg	Potassium mg	Vit A %rda	Vit B1 %rda (thiamin)	Vit B2 %rda (riboflavin)	Vit B3 %rda (niacin)	Vit C %rda	Calcium %rda	Iron %rda
Lard	1 tb	115	0	13	0	0	0	0	0	0	0	0	0	0	0
Margarine, soft	1 tb	100	0	12	0	0	140	4	*	0	0	*	0	*	0
Margarine, stick	1 tb	102	0	12	0	0	140	4	*	*	0	*	0	0	0
Margarine, whipped	1 tb	70	0	8	0	0	93	2	*	0	0	*	0	*	0
Olive oil	1 tb	120	0	14	0	0	0	NA	0	0	0	0	0	0	0
Peanut oil	1 tb	120	0	14	0	0	0	NA	0	0	0	0	0	0	0
Safflower oil	1 tb	120	0	14	0	0	0	NA	0	0	0	0	0	0	0
Shortening, vegetable	1 tb	110	0	13	0	0	0	NA	0	0	0	0	0	0	0
Soybean oil	1 tb	120	0	14	0	0	0	NA	0	0	0	0	0	0	0

Miscellaneous

Food	Serving	Calories	Protein g	Fat g	Carbo g	Fiber g	Sodium mg	Potassium mg	Vit A %rda	Vit B1 %rda (thiamin)	Vit B2 %rda (riboflavin)	Vit B3 %rda (niacin)	Vit C %rda	Calcium %rda	Iron %rda
Baking powder	1 ts	5	0	0	1	0	349	NA	0	0	0	0	0	18	NA
Baking powder, low-sodium	1 ts	5	0	0	2	0	1	471	0	0	0	0	0	21	NA
Chocolate, baking	1 oz	145	3	15	8	0	1	235	1	1	4	2	0	2	11
Cocoa powder	1 tb	14	1	1	3	0	1	0	*	1	1	1	1	1	3
Cornstarch	1 tb	29	0	0	7	0	1	1	0	0	0	0	0	0	0
Gelatin, dry	1 pk	25	6	0	0	0	NA	NA	NA	NA	NA	NA	NA	NA	0
Vinegar	1 tb	0	0	0	1	0	0	15	NA	NA	NA	NA	0	1	1
Yeast, baker's	1 pk	20	3	0	3	1	1	140	*	11	13	*	0	6	6
Yeast, brewer's	1 tb	25	3	0	3	3	10	152	*	83	20	15	*	2	8

Salad Dressings

Food	Serving	Calories	Protein g	Fat g	Carbo g	Fiber g	Sodium mg	Potassium mg	Vit A %rda	Vit B1 %rda (thiamin)	Vit B2 %rda (riboflavin)	Vit B3 %rda (niacin)	Vit C %rda	Calcium %rda	Iron %rda
Bacon & tomato Kraft	1 tb	70	0	7	0	0	130	NA	*	*	*	*	*	*	*
Blue cheese, chunky Wish-Bone	1 tb	70	0	7	1	0	150	NA	*	*	*	*	*	*	*
Buttermilk, creamy Kraft	1 tb	80	0	8	1	0	120	NA	*	*	*	*	*	*	*
Buttermilk, creamy, lo-cal, Kraft	1 tb	30	0	3	1	0	125	NA	*	*	*	*	*	*	*
California onion Wish-Bone	1 tb	70	0	8	1	0	155	NA	*	*	*	*	*	*	*
Creamy garlic Wish-Bone	1 tb	80	0	8	2	0	170	NA	*	*	*	*	*	*	*
Cucumber, creamy Kraft	1 tb	70	0	8	1	0	200	NA	*	*	*	*	*	*	*
Cucumber, creamy, lo-cal, Kraft	1 tb	30	0	3	1	0	230	NA	*	*	*	*	*	*	*
Deluxe French Wish-Bone	1 tb	60	0	5	3	0	75	NA	*	NA	NA	NA	*	*	*
French, low-cal	1 tb	15	0	1	2	0	126	13	NA	NA	NA	NA	0	1	0
French, sweet 'n spicy, Wish-bone	1 tb	60	0	5	3	0	150	NA	*	*	*	*	*	*	*

Salad Dressings, cont'd.

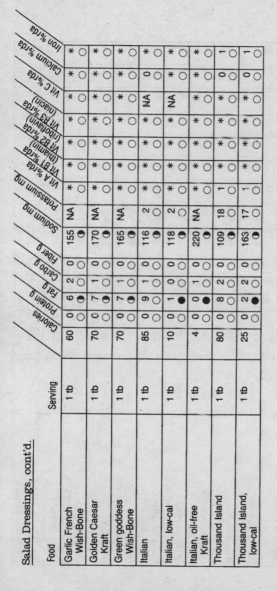

Food	Serving	Calories	Protein g	Fat g	Carbo g	Fiber g	Sodium mg	Potassium mg	Vit A %rda	Vit B1 %rda (thiamin)	Vit B2 %rda (riboflavin)	Vit B3 %rda (niacin)	Vit C %rda	Calcium %rda	Iron %rda
Garlic French Wish-Bone	1 tb	60	0	6	2	0	155	NA	*	*	*	*	*	*	*
Golden Caesar Kraft	1 tb	70	0	7	1	0	170	NA	*	*	*	*	*	*	*
Green goddess Wish-Bone	1 tb	70	0	7	1	0	165	NA	*	*	*	*	*	*	*
Italian	1 tb	85	0	9	1	0	116	2	*	*	*	NA	*	*	*
Italian, low-cal	1 tb	10	0	1	0	0	118	2	*	*	*	NA	*	*	*
Italian, oil-free Kraft	1 tb	4	0	0	1	0	220	NA	*	*	*	*	*	*	*
Thousand Island	1 tb	80	0	8	2	0	109	18	1	*	*	*	*	1	1
Thousand Island, low-cal	1 tb	25	0	2	2	0	163	17	1	*	*	*	*	1	1

Sauces

Food	Serving	Calories	Protein g	Fat g	Carbo g	Fiber g	Sodium mg	Potassium mg	Vit A %rda	Vit B1 %rda (thiamin)	Vit B2 %rda (riboflavin)	Vit B3 %rda (niacin)	Vit C %rda	Calcium %rda	Iron %rda
Barbecue, Kraft	¼ c	90 ○	0 ○	2 ●	18 ●	0 ○	990 ○	16 ○	* ○	* ○	* ○	* ○	* ○	* ○	* ○
Barbecue, hickory Kraft	¼ c	80 ○	0 ○	2 ●	18 ●	0 ○	970 ○	16 ○	* ○	* ○	* ○	* ○	* ○	4 ○	* ○
Barbecue, hot Kraft	¼ c	80 ○	0 ○	2 ●	16 ●	0 ○	1240 ○	12 ○	* ○	* ○	* ○	* ○	* ○	4 ○	* ○
Cheese, from mix French's	¼ c	80 ○	3 ○	4 ●	7 ●	0 ○	425 ○	* ○	* ○	* ○	8 ○	* ○	10 ●	* ○	* ○
Gravy for pork, from mix, French's	¼ c	20 ○	1 ○	1 ●	3 ○	0 ○	280 ●	* ○	* ○	* ○	* ○	* ○	* ○	* ○	* ○
Gravy for turkey, from mix, French's	¼ c	25 ○	1 ○	1 ●	4 ○	0 ○	380 ●	* ○	* ○	* ○	* ○	* ○	* ○	* ○	* ○
Gravy, au jus, from mix, French's	¼ c	8 ○	0 ○	0 ●	2 ○	0 ○	265 ●	* ○	* ○	* ○	* ○	* ○	* ○	* ○	* ○
Gravy, beef Franco-American	¼ c	25 ○	1 ○	2 ●	3 ○	0 ○	330 ○	* ○	* ○	* ○	* ○	* ○	* ○	* ○	* ○
Gravy, brown, from mix, French's	¼ c	20 ○	1 ○	1 ●	3 ○	0 ○	280 ●	* ○	* ○	* ○	* ○	* ○	* ○	* ○	* ○
Gravy, chicken Franco-American	¼ c	50 ○	0 ○	4 ●	3 ○	0 ○	320 ●	2 ○	* ○	* ○	* ○	* ○	* ○	* ○	* ○
Gravy, mushroom Franco-American	¼ c	25 ○	1 ●	1 ●	3 ○	0 ○	320 ●	* ○	* ○	* ○	* ○	* ○	* ○	* ○	* ○

Sodium mg column also shows: NA

Sauces, cont'd.

Food	Serving	Calories	Protein g	Fat g	Carbo g	Fiber g	Sodium mg	Potassium mg	Vit A %rda	Vit B1 %rda (thiamin)	Vit B2 %rda (riboflavin)	Vit B3 %rda (niacin)	Vit C %rda	Calcium %rda	Iron %rda
Gravy, onion, from mix, French's	¼ c	25	1	1	4	0	350	NA	*	*	*	*	*	*	*
Hollandaise, from mix, French's	¼ c	59	1	5	3	0	386	NA	*	*	3	*	3	*	*
Pizza, Contadina	½ c	80	2	4	10	0	700	395	20	4	4	15	2	6	8
Pizza, w/cheese Contadina	½ c	90	2	4	11	0	750	459	25	4	4	20	4	4	8
Pizza, w/pepperoni Contadina	½ c	80	2	4	9	0	715	428	25	4	4	20	2	4	8
Prima Salsa, meat flavor	½ c	120	4	3	20	0	NA	NA	30	6	8	20	*	2	8
Prima Salsa, regular or mushroom	½ c	110	3	3	20	0	NA	NA	30	6	8	20	*	2	8
Sour cream, from mix, French's	¼ c	96	3	8	8	0	208	*	*	*	6	*	10	*	*
Spaghetti, Italian from mix, French's	½ c	80	2	3	12	0	720	NA	28	5	3	24	2	6	5
Spaghetti, thick, from mix French's	½ c	97	2	4	14	0	831	NA	29	6	3	29	1	6	5

Sauces, cont'd.

Food	Serving	Calories	Protein g	Fat g	Carbo g	Fiber g	Sodium mg	Potassium mg	Vit A %rda	Vit B1 %rda (thiamin)	Vit B2 %rda (riboflavin)	Vit B3 %rda (niacin)	Vit C %rda	Calcium %rda	Iron %rda
Stroganoff, from mix, French's	¼ c	82	4	4	8	0	367	NA	2	6	5	*	*	8	*
Sweet & sour La Choy	¼ c	131	0	0	32	0	320	NA	NA	NA	NA	NA	NA	NA	NA
Sweet 'n sour Contadina	¼ c	60	1	1	13	0	225	66	*	1	*	2	2	*	1
Swiss steak Contadina	¼ c	20	1	0	5	0	319	171	1	2	5	2	2	2	2
Teriyaki, from mix French's	¼ c	70	2	0	14	0	2360	NA	*	*	*	*	*	4	8
Tomato paste w/mushrooms Contadina	2 oz	60	2	1	12	NA	550	450	20	4	4	8	20	2	4
Tomato paste, Hunt	¼ c	52	2	0	11	NA	168	30	30	6	6	8	38	2	5
Tomato, Contadina	½ c	45	2	0	9	NA	680	537	25	2	6	6	15	*	4
Tomato, Hunt	½ c	35	1	0	8	NA	665	20	20	4	6	6	10	*	2
Tomato, herb, Hunt	½ c	80	2	4	12	NA	495	20	20	6	6	6	15	2	4

Sauces, cont'd.

Food	Serving	Calories	Protein g	Fat g	Carbo g	Fiber g	Sodium mg	Potassium mg	Vit A % rda	Vit B1 % rda (thiamin)	Vit B2 % rda (riboflavin)	Vit B3 % rda (niacin)	Vit C % rda	Calcium % rda	Iron % rda
Tomato, special Hunt	½ c	40	1	0 ●	10 ●	NA	NA	NA	15	4	4	6	15	*	2
Tomato, w/bits Hunt	½ c	35	1	0	8	NA	695	NA	20	4	4	6	20 ●	*	2
Tomato, w/cheese Hunt	½ c	70	3	2 ●	10 ●	NA	795	NA	20	4	6	8	10	4	4
Tomato, w/mushrooms Hunt	½ c	40	1	0	9 ●	NA	710	NA	20	4	4	8	25 ●	*	4
White, medium	¼ c	101	3	6	0	0	87 ●	87	6	2	6	1	1	7	1

Combination Foods
Breakfasts, Frozen

Food	Serving	Calories	Protein g	Fat g	Carbo g	Fiber g	Sodium mg	Potassium mg	Vit A % rda	Vit B1 % rda (thiamin)	Vit B2 % rda (riboflavin)	Vit B3 % rda (niacin)	Vit C % rda	Calcium % rda	Iron % rda
French toast Downyflake	2 sl	270	4	14	30	NA	NA	NA	*	10	10	10	*	8	10
French toast w/sausage Hungry-Man	1	270	12	28	NA	NA	665	NA	*	25	20	15	*	8	10
Omelets w/ham & cheese sauce Hungry-Man	1	400	19	32	11	NA	1305	15	8	8	25	4	25	10	10
Pancakes w/blueberries Hungry-Man	1	400	9	9	70	NA	740	NA	20	20	20	10	6	10	10
Pancakes w/sausage Hungry-Man	1	440	16	24	48	NA	985	NA	35	35	20	20	6	10	10
Scrambled eggs w/sausage Hungry-Man	1	430	13	35	17	NA	730	NA	10	10	20	8	4	10	10

Entrees, Frozen

Food	Serving	Calories	Protein g	Fat g	Carbo g	Fiber g	Sodium mg	Potassium mg	Vit A %rda	Vit B1 %rda (thiamin)	Vit B2 %rda (riboflavin)	Vit B3 %rda (niacin)	Vit C %rda	Calcium %rda	Iron %rda
Asparagus souffle, 12 oz, Stouffers	1/3	115	6 ●	7 ●	8	NA ○	440 ○	190 ○	10 ●	6 ○	10 ●	2 ○	* ○	8 ○	4 ○
Beef pie, Hungry-Man	1	720	30 ●	38 ○	65 ●	NA	1490 ○	NA	25 ◐	30 ●	35 ●	30 ●	10 ○	2 ○	25 ●
Beef stew & biscuits, Green Giant	7 oz	190	14 ●	6 ●	21 ●	NA	NA	NA	20 ●	8 ○	8 ○	8 ○	15 ○	4 ○	10 ●
Beef strogonoff, 9.8 oz, Stouffers	1	390	22 ●	20 ●	31 ●	NA	1300 ●	320 ●	4 ○	20 ●	15 ●	25 ●	* ○	4 ○	20 ●
Cheese souffle, 12 oz, Stouffers	1/2	355	18 ●	26 ○	14 ●	NA	1360 ○	275 ●	15 ○	10 ●	25 ●	2 ○	* ○	30 ●	8 ○
Chicken & biscuits, Green Giant	7 oz	200	17 ●	6 ●	19 ●	NA	NA	NA	25 ●	4 ○	6 ○	25 ●	15 ○	8 ○	2 ○
Chicken ala king, 9.5 oz, Stouffers	1	330	21 ●	11 ●	38 ●	NA	900 ●	280 ●	4 ○	6 ○	10 ●	25 ●	* ○	10 ○	8 ○
Chicken divan, 8.5 oz, Stouffers	1	335	21 ●	22 ○	14 ●	NA	830 ●	415 ●	35 ●	10 ○	15 ○	20 ●	15 ○	20 ●	6 ○
Chicken pie, Hungry-Man	1	730	28 ●	39 ●	65 ●	NA	1680 ●	NA	60 ●	25 ●	25 ●	40 ●	10 ○	* ○	20 ●
Crabs, devilled, Mrs Paul's	1 pc	170	8 ●	8 ○	17 ●	NA	510 ○	NA	6 ○	8 ○	10 ●	10 ●	0 ○	10 ●	6 ○

Entrees, Frozen, cont'd.

Food	Serving	Calories	Protein g	Fat g	Carbo g	Fiber g	Sodium mg	Potassium mg	Vit A %rda	Vit B1 %rda (thiamin)	Vit B2 %rda (riboflavin)	Vit B3 %rda (niacin)	Vit C %rda	Calcium %rda	Iron %rda
Crepe, chicken, 8.2 oz, Stouffers	1	390	30 ●	22	19	NA	1040 ●	420 ●	8 ○	10 ●	25 ●	25 ●	* ○	15 ○	8 ○
Crepe, mushroom, 6.3 oz, Stouffers	1	255	10 ●	13	27	NA	865 ●	325 ●	6 ○	10 ●	35 ●	15 ●	* ○	6 ○	8 ○
Crepe, beef burgundy, 6.3 oz, Stouffers	1	335	23 ●	17 ○	24 ●	NA	830 ○	465 ●	10 ○	10 ●	20 ●	25 ●	* ○	8 ○	15 ●
Crepe, spinach, 9.5 oz, Stouffers	1	415	16 ●	25 ●	30	NA	995 ○	440 ●	50 ○	10 ●	40 ●	6 ○	* ○	30 ●	25 ●
Eggplant parmigiana, 16 oz, Celentano	½	304	10 ●	19 ○	19	NA	NA	NA	36 ●	*	12 ●	34 ●	10	24 ●	22 ●
Fish parmesan, 10 oz, Mrs Paul's	½	220	11 ●	11 ○	20 ●	NA	1000 ○	NA	10 ○	8	6 ○	15 ●	4 ○	4 ○	2 ○
Lobster newburg, 6.5 oz, Stouffers	1	350	15 ●	29 ○	9	NA	700 ○	190 ○	20 ●	2	20 ●	4	* ○	10 ○	6 ○
Macaroni & cheese, 12 oz, Stouffers	½	260	12 ●	24 ●	24	NA	780 ○	140 ○	4 ○	10	10 ●	4	* ○	25 ●	6 ○
Spinach souffle, Green Giant	1 c	300	10 ●	17 ○	27	NA	NA	NA	30 ○	8 ○	30 ●	2 ○	15 ●	25 ●	10 ●
Spinach souffle, 12 oz, Stouffers	⅓	135	5 ○	7 ●	12	NA	600 ●	250 ●	8 ○	8	8 ○	2	* ○	8 ○	8 ○
Steak burger pie, Hungry-Man	1	760	27 ●	46 ●	61 ●	NA	1460 ○	NA	40 ●	25 ●	30 ●	35 ●	10	4 ○	25 ●

Entrees, Frozen, cont'd.

Food	Serving	Calories	Protein g	Fat g	Carbo g	Fiber g	Sodium mg	Potassium mg	Vit A %rda	Vit B1 %rda (thiamin)	Vit B2 %rda (riboflavin)	Vit B3 %rda (niacin)	Vit C %rda	Calcium %rda	Iron %rda
Steak, green pepper 10.5 oz, Stouffers	1	350 ●	25 ●	13 ○	35 ●	NA	1500 ○	430 ●	8 ○	4 ○	15 ●	25 ●	* ○	2 ○	15 ●
Stuffed cabbage w/beef Green Giant	7 oz	220 ○	10 ●	12 ○	17 ●	NA	820 ○	NA	35 ●	4 ○	4 ○	10 ●	20 ●	2 ○	8 ○
Stuffed pepper, 15 oz, Stouffers	½	225 ●	10 ●	11 ○	18 ●	NA	960 ○	420 ●	10 ●	10 ●	8 ○	20 ●	* ○	4 ○	10 ●
Stuffed potato w/cheese topping Green Giant	5 oz	240 ●	4 ●	12 ○	30 ●	NA	NA	NA	* ○	* ○	4 ○	6 ○	10 ○	4 ○	6 ○
Swedish meatballs, 11 oz, Stouffers	1	475 ●	25 ●	27 ○	33 ●	NA	1620 ○	395 ●	10 ○	15 ●	20 ●	25 ●	* ○	8 ●	25 ●
Tuna noodle casserole, 11.5 oz Stouffers	½	200 ●	10 ●	9 ○	18 ●	NA	670 ○	210 ●	10 ●	10 ●	10 ●	15 ●	* ○	10 ●	6 ○
Turkey Tetrazzini, 12 oz, Stouffers	½	240 ●	12 ●	14 ○	17 ●	NA	620 ○	200 ○	* ○	10 ●	10 ●	10 ○	* ○	8 ○	8 ○
Welsh rarebit, 10 oz, Stouffers	½	355 ●	8 ●	29 ○	17 ●	NA	660 ○	155 ○	20 ○	6 ○	15 ●	* ○	40 ●	40 ●	2 ○

Ethnic Dishes

Food	Serving	Calories	Protein g	Fat g	Carbo g	Fiber g	Sodium mg	Potassium mg	Vit A % rda	Vit B1 % rda (thiamin)	Vit B2 % rda (riboflavin)	Vit B3 % rda (niacin)	Vit C % rda	Calcium % rda	Iron % rda
Beans, refried Old El Paso	½ c	100	7 ●	1 ●	17	NA	NA	NA	* ○	2 ○	2 ○	2 ○	* ○	6 ○	10 ●
Beans, refried w/green chilies Old El Paso	½ c	92	6 ●	0 ●	16	NA	279 ●	330 ●	* ○	4 ○	4 ○	* ○	* ○	4 ○	10 ●
Beans, refried w/sausage Olc El Paso	½ c	194	7 ●	13 ○	13	NA	312 ●	300 ●	* ○	2 ○	4 ○	2 ○	* ○	4 ○	10 ●
Borscht, diet Rokeach	1 c	29	1 ○	0 ●	6	NA	897 ○	* ○	* ○	* ○	2 ○	13 ○	* ○	* ○	* ○
Borscht, regular Rokeach	1 c	96	1 ○	0 ●	1	NA	985 ○	* ○	* ○	* ○	3 ○	13 ○	* ○	* ○	* ○
Borscht, unsalted Rokeach	1 c	102	1 ○	0 ●	24	NA	50 ●	* ○	* ○	* ○	2 ○	13 ○	* ○	* ○	* ○
Burrito, bean & cheese, 5 oz Pinata	1	310	13 ●	9 ○	45 ●	NA	523 ○	4 ○	20 ●	10 ●	10 ●	1 ○	15 ●	10 ●	10 ●
Burrito, beef & bean, 5 oz Pinata	1	330	12 ○	12 ○	43 ●	NA	515 ●	8 ○	20 ●	10 ●	10 ●	1 ○	10 ●	10 ●	10 ●

Ethnic Dishes, cont'd.

Food	Serving	Calories	Protein g	Fat g	Carbo g	Fiber g	Sodium mg	Potassium mg	Vit A %rda	Vit B1 %rda (thiamin)	Vit B2 %rda (riboflavin)	Vit B3 %rda (niacin)	Vit C %rda	Calcium %rda	Iron %rda
Burrito, green chili, 5 oz Pinata	1	320 ●	12 ●	14 ●	37 ●	NA	623 ○	6 ○	20 ●	10 ●	10 ●	10 ●	10 ●	10 ●	10 ●
Burrito, red chili, 5 oz, Pinata	1	330 ●	12 ●	12 ○	43 ●	NA	550 ○	8 ○	20 ●	10 ●	10 ●	10 ●	10 ●	10 ●	10 ●
Chili w/beans, 15 oz Chef Boyardee	½ cn	330 ●	15 ●	17 ○	30 ●	NA	1005 ○	20 ○	6 ○	8 ○	10 ●	10 ●	6 ○	20 ●	20 ●
Chili w/o beans, 15 oz Chef Boyardee	½ cn	370 ●	14 ●	29 ○	14 ○	NA	875 ○	30 ○	2 ○	10 ●	20 ●	6 ○	2 ○	10 ●	10 ●
Chilies, green Old El Paso	3.5 oz	25 ○	1 ○	0 ●	5 ○	NA	NA	* ○	* ○	* ○	* ○	70 ●	10 ●	4 ○	4 ○
Chow mein, beef, canned, La Choy	1 c	72 ○	7 ●	2 ●	6 ○	NA	976 ○	NA	NA	NA	NA	NA	NA	NA	NA
Chow mein, chicken, canned, La Choy	1 c	68 ○	7 ●	2 ●	5 ○	NA	924 ○	NA	NA	NA	NA	NA	NA	NA	NA
Chow mein, meatless canned, La Choy	1 c	47 ○	3 ○	1 ●	6 ○	NA	835 ○	NA	NA	NA	NA	NA	NA	NA	NA
Chow mein, mushroom canned, La Choy	1 c	85 ○	3 ○	3 ●	11 ●	NA	1161 ○	NA	NA	NA	NA	NA	NA	NA	NA

Ethnic Dishes, cont'd.

Food	Serving	Calories	Protein g	Fat g	Carbo g	Fiber g	Sodium mg	Potassium mg	Vit A %rda	Vit B1 %rda (thiamin)	Vit B2 %rda (riboflavin)	Vit B3 %rda (niacin)	Vit C %rda	Calcium %rda	Iron %rda
Chow mein, pork, canned, La Choy	1 c	120	6	6	11	NA	1675	NA	NA	NA	NA	NA	NA	NA	NA
Chow mein, shrimp, canned, La Choy	1 c	61	6	2	6	NA	951	NA	NA	NA	NA	NA	NA	NA	NA
Egg roll, shrimp La Choy	1	108	5	3	15	NA	393	NA	NA	NA	NA	NA	NA	NA	NA
Fritters, apple Mrs Paul's	2 pc	240	3	12	32	NA	1080	NA	0	12	0	8	0	4	4
Fritters, corn Mrs Paul's	2 pc	260	6	12	31	NA	1520	NA	2	4	15	2	0	2	2
Gefilte fish, Redi-Jelled Rokeach	1 pc	92	12	2	6	0	444	NA	*	7	3	6	6	3	3
Gefilte fish, natural broth Rokeach	1 pc	50	7	1	4	0	NA	NA	*	4	*	2	4	*	*
Matzo, American Manischewitz	1	115	3	2	22	NA	NA	NA	NA	NA	NA	NA	*	NA	NA
Matzo, egg 'n onion Manischewitz	1	112	3	1	22	NA	NA	NA	11	6	5	*	*	6	6
Matzo, unsalted Manischewitz	1	112	3	0	24	1	34	NA	9	5	6	*	*	5	5

Ethnic Dishes, cont'd.

Food	Serving	Calories	Protein g	Fat g	Carbo g	Fiber g	Sodium mg	Potassium mg	Vit A %rda	Vit B1 %rda (thiamin)	Vit B2 %rda (riboflavin)	Vit B3 %rda (niacin)	Vit C %rda	Calcium %rda	Iron %rda
Matzo, whole wheat w/bran, Manischewitz	1	110	4	1	22	1	1	NA	*	7	4	*	*	8	8
Okra gumbo Green Giant	1 c	220	2	18	12	NA	NA	NA	8	4	4	50	6	4	4
Pierogies, potato & cheese Mrs Paul's	3	300	10	4	56	NA	550	NA	15	15	20	2	2	6	6
Pierogies, sauerkraut Mrs Paul's	3	310	9	3	60	NA	400	0	25	15	15	2	2	10	10
Pierogies, cabbage Mrs Paul's	3	330	9	4	63	NA	650	0	30	15	10	2	2	8	8
Pig's feet, pickled	2 oz	113	10	8	0	0	NA	NA	NA	NA	NA	NA	NA	NA	NA
Ramen, beef La Choy	1 c	225	6	8	33	NA	NA	NA	NA	NA	NA	NA	NA	NA	NA
Ramen, chicken La Choy	1 c	202	6	7	29	NA	NA	NA	NA	NA	NA	NA	NA	NA	NA
Taco shell Old El Paso	1	51	1	2	7	NA	50	*	4	4	2	*	*	2	2

Ethnic Dishes, cont'd.

Food	Serving	Calories	Protein g	Fat g	Carbo g	Fiber g	Sodium mg	Potassium mg	Vit A %rda	Vit B1 %rda (thiamin)	Vit B2 %rda (riboflavin)	Vit B3 %rda (niacin)	Vit C %rda	Calcium %rda	Iron %rda
Tamales Old El Paso	2	232	6	13	23	NA	NA	NA	2	*	8	8	*	3	25
Tomatoes & green chilies Old El Paso	3.5 oz	23	1	0	4	NA	487	248	*	*	3	5	12	*	4
Whitefish-pike Rokeach	1 pc	60	9	1	4	NA	NA	NA	2	*	4	2	8	4	*
Wonton soup La Choy	1 c	92	6	2	12	NA	2027	NA	NA	NA	NA	NA	NA	NA	NA

Pasta Entrees

Food	Serving	Calories	Protein g	Fat g	Carbo g	Fiber g	Sodium mg	Potassium mg	Vit A %rda	Vit B1 %rda (thiamin)	Vit B2 %rda (riboflavin)	Vit B3 %rda (niacin)	Vit C %rda	Calcium %rda	Iron %rda
Fettucine Alfredo, 10 oz Stouffers	½	270	8	18	19	NA	1194	237	6	10	4	*	15	2	
Lasagne, 16 oz Celentano	½	354	17	15	38	NA	738	NA	12	25	15	19	20	16	
Linguini, w/clam sauce, 10.5 oz Stouffers	1	285	17	8	36	NA	1010	115	20	10	10	*	2	15	

Pasta Entrees, cont'd.

Food	Serving	Calories	Protein g	Fat g	Carbo g	Fiber g	Sodium mg	Potassium mg	Vit A %rda	Vit B1 %rda (thiamin)	Vit B2 %rda (riboflavin)	Vit B3 %rda (niacin)	Vit C %rda	Calcium %rda	Iron %rda
Macaroni & cheese Franco-American	1 cn	170	6	6	24	NA	960	NA	6	15	10	8	*	8	6
Macaroni & cheese Kraft	¾ c	300	8	14	36	NA	625	NA	10	15	15	8	*	8	10
Manicotti, 16 oz Celentano	½	322	15	13	35	NA	720	NA	22	33	15	18	18	21	18
Ravioli, 13 oz Celentano	½	426	21	15	52	NA	562	NA	8	35	18	*	*	23	22
Ravioli, beef Chef Boyardee	½ cn	200	7	6	31	NA	1233	NA	10	6	10	10	*	*	10
Ravioli, beef w/meat sauce Franco-American	1 cn	230	9	5	36	NA	1170	NA	8	8	10	10	4	2	10
Ravioli, cheese, 15 oz Chef Boyardee	½ cn	200	7	5	33	NA	1116	NA	8	10	10	10	*	6	10
RavioliO, cheese	1 cn	260	7	8	39	NA	1160	NA	6	8	10	10	2	10	8
Spaghetti & meatball, 15 oz Chef Boyardee	½ cn	230	7	11	26	NA	1052	NA	6	10	10	10	*	*	10

Pasta Entrees, cont'd.

Food	Serving	Calories	Protein g	Fat g	Carbo g	Fiber g	Sodium mg	Potassium mg	Vit A %rda	Vit B1 %rda (thiamin)	Vit B2 %rda (riboflavin)	Vit B3 %rda (niacin)	Vit C %rda	Calcium %rda	Iron %rda
Spaghetti w/meat sauce Franco-American	1 cn	220	8 ●	9 ○	26 ●	NA	1130 ○	NA	10 ○	10 ○	10 ●	15 ●	4 ○	2 ○	10 ●
Spaghetti w/meatballs Franco-American	1 cn	220	9 ●	8 ○	27 ●	NA	1040 ○	NA	10 ○	8 ○	8 ○	15 ●	4 ○	2 ○	10 ●
Spaghetti w/tomato sauce & cheese Franco-American	1 cn	180	5 ●	2 ○	36 ●	NA	940 ○	NA	15 ●	8 ○	8 ○	10 ●	* ○	2 ○	6 ○
Spaghetti w/tomato sauce&cheese, 15 oz Chef Boyardee	½ cn	150	4 ●	1 ●	31 ●	NA	1040 ○	NA	6 ○	6 ○	6 ○	8 ○	* ○	2 ○	6 ○

Pizza, Frozen

Food	Serving	Calories	Protein g	Fat g	Carbo g	Fiber g	Sodium mg	Potassium mg	Vit A %rda	Vit B1 %rda (thiamin)	Vit B2 %rda (riboflavin)	Vit B3 %rda (niacin)	Vit C %rda	Calcium %rda	Iron %rda
Cheese, 10.3 oz Stouffers	½	330	10 ●	13 ○	43 ●	NA	850 ●	220 ●	25 ●	10 ●	15 ●	* ○	25 ●	15 ●	6 ●
Cheese, 13 oz Chef Boyardee	½	360	19 ●	9 ○	51 ●	NA	925 ●	NA	30 ●	25 ●	20 ●	* ○	30 ●	15 ●	6 ○
Cheese, 19 oz Celeste	¼	310	16 ●	13 ○	32 ●	NA	805 ●	260 ●	6 ○	20 ●	6 ○	* ○	35 ●	6 ○	6 ○

Pizza, Frozen, cont'd.

Food	Serving	Calories	Protein g	Fat g	Carbo g	Fiber g	Sodium mg	Potassium mg	Vit A %rda	Vit B1 %rda (thiamin)	Vit B2 %rda (riboflavin)	Vit B3 %rda (niacin)	Vit C %rda	Calcium %rda	Iron %rda
Deluxe, 12.4 oz Stouffers	½	400	15●	18●	46	NA	1150	325○	15○	20●	20●	20●	*○	20●	15●
Deluxe, 15.5 oz Chef Boyardee	½	430	21●	16○	51●	NA	1135○	NA	10○	35●	25●	25●	2○	25●	20●
Deluxe, 24 oz Celeste	¼	370	17●	17○	38●	NA	1050○	425●	15○	20●	30●	10◐	*○	25●	8○
Hamburger, 12.3 oz Stouffers	½	400	17●	20○	39●	NA	1100○	265○	15○	20●	20●	15●	*○	20●	15●
Pepperoni, 20 oz Celeste	¼	350	17●	16○	35●	NA	1080○	255○	20○	15●	35●	10●	*○	30●	6●
Pizza, thick-crust, 13 oz Celentano	⅓	238	13●	7◐	31●	NA	NA	252●	12○	14◐	16◐	11◐	5○	9○	7○
Sausage, 14 oz Chef Boyardee	½	430	20●	16○	51●	NA	1170○	NA	15○	35●	25●	25●	*○	30●	15●
Sausage, 22 oz Celeste	¼	360	18●	17○	35●	NA	1225○	275○	20○	15●	35●	10●	*○	30●	8○
Suprema, 24 oz Celeste	¼	360	19●	32○	17◐	NA	NA	NA	6○	15●	25●	10●	*○	30●	10●

Soups, Prep As Directed

Food	Serving	Calories	Protein g	Fat g	Carbo g	Fiber g	Sodium mg	Potassium mg	Vit A %rda	Vit B1 %rda (thiamin)	Vit B2 %rda (riboflavin)	Vit B3 %rda (niacin)	Vit C %rda	Calcium %rda	Iron %rda
Bean w/bacon Campbell	1 c	150	6	5	21	NA	990	10	4	*	2	*	6	6	8
Beef Campbell	1 c	80	5	2	10	NA	950	15	*	2	4	2	*	*	2
Beef noodle Campbell	1 c	70	4	3	7	NA	990	2	4	2	4	*	*	*	4
Black bean Campbell	1 c	110	5	2	17	NA	1125	4	*	*	*	*	2	2	10
Bouillon cube	1	5	1	0	0	NA	960	4	NA	NA	NA	NA	NA	NA	NA
Chicken gumbo Campbell	1 c	60	2	2	8	NA	930	*	*	*	2	*	*	*	2
Chicken noodle Campbell	1 c	70	3	2	8	NA	960	4	4	2	4	2	*	*	4
Chicken noodle, low-sodium Campbell	1 cn	90	4	4	9	NA	40	10	10	6	10	*	*	4	4
Chicken w/rice Campbell	1 c	60	2	3	7	NA	890	*	*	*	2	*	*	*	*
Chunky bean w/ham Campbell	½ cn	250	12	9	32	NA	1220	80	8	8	8	6	8	8	15

Soups, Prep As Directed, cont'd.

Food	Serving	Calories	Protein g	Fat g	Carbo g	Fiber g	Sodium mg	Potassium mg	Vit A %rda	Vit B1 %rda (thiamin)	Vit B2 %rda (riboflavin)	Vit B3 %rda (niacin)	Vit C %rda	Calcium %rda	Iron %rda
Chunky beef, Campbell	½ cn	170	13 ●	4 ●	20 ●	NA	1130 ○	80 ●	2 ○	8 ○	10 ○	10 ○	2 ○	10 ●	10 ●
Chunky beef-mushroom, low-sodium, Campbell	1 cn	200	12 ●	7 ●	23 ●	NA	75 ●	60 ●	8 ○	20 ●	20 ●	6 ○	2 ○	15 ●	15 ●
Chunky chicken, Campbell	½ cn	180	12 ●	7 ●	18 ●	NA	1130 ○	15 ○	6 ○	10 ●	20 ●	* ○	2 ○	8 ○	8 ○
Chunky chicken, low-sodium, Campbell	1 cn	150	10 ●	6 ●	14 ●	NA	70 ●	10 ○	6 ○	10 ●	15 ●	* ○	2 ○	6 ○	6 ●
Chunky pea w/ham, Campbell	½ cn	200	11 ●	5 ●	29 ●	NA	1210 ○	50 ●	4 ○	4 ○	10 ●	10 ○	2 ○	8 ○	8 ○
Chunky sirloin, Campbell	½ cn	200	11 ●	8 ○	20 ●	NA	1250 ○	60 ●	* ○	8 ○	10 ●	10 ○	2 ○	10 ●	10 ●
Chunky turkey, Campbell	½ cn	180	9 ●	7 ●	18 ●	NA	1290 ○	140 ●	2 ○	6 ○	10 ●	6 ○	2 ○	6 ○	6 ○
Chunky vegetable, Campbell	½ cn	130	3 ○	4 ●	21 ●	NA	1300 ○	120 ●	* ○	2 ○	4 ○	10 ●	4 ○	4 ○	4 ○
Clam chowder, Manhattan, Campbell	1 c	70	2 ○	2 ●	11 ●	NA	940 ○	30 ●	* ○	* ○	2 ○	8 ○	2 ○	2 ○	2 ○

Soups, Prep As Directed, cont'd.

Food	Serving	Calories	Protein g	Fat g	Carbo g	Fiber g	Sodium mg	Potassium mg	Vit A %rda	Vit B1 %rda (thiamin)	Vit B2 %rda (riboflavin)	Vit B3 %rda (niacin)	Vit C %rda	Calcium %rda	Iron %rda
Clam chowder, New England Campbell	1 c	80	3	3	11	NA	965	NA	*	*	*	2	2	2	2
Cream of celery Campbell	1 c	100	1	7	8	NA	940	4	*	*	*	*	2	2	*
Cream of chicken Campbell	1 c	110	3	7	9	NA	950	10	*	*	2	2	2	2	*
Cream of mushroom Campbell	1 c	100	1	7	9	NA	870	*	*	*	2	2	*	*	*
Cream of mushroom, low-sodium Campbell	1 cn	130	1	9	10	NA	35	*	*	*	4	2	2	2	2
Cream of potato Campbell	1 c	70	1	3	11	NA	960	2	*	*	*	*	*	*	*
Cup-a-soup, chicken vegetable	¾ c	40	2	1	7	NA	761	15	*	*	2	2	*	2	2
Cup-a-soup, country style Virginia pea	¾ c	140	5	5	18	NA	NA	*	40	2	2	*	*	2	*
Cup-a-soup, country style chicken supreme	¾ c	100	3	5	11	NA	NA	*	2	2	2	*	2	2	2

Soups, Prep As Directed, cont'd.

Food	Serving	Calories	Protein g	Fat g	Carbo g	Fiber g	Sodium mg	Potassium mg	Vit A %rda	Vit B1 %rda (thiamin)	Vit B2 %rda (riboflavin)	Vit B3 %rda (niacin)	Vit C %rda	Calcium %rda	Iron %rda
Cup-a-soup, country style harvest vegetable	¾ c	100	2○	1●	20●	NA	NA	25●	4○	4○	2○	4○	*○	2○	4○
Cup-a-soup, country style hearty chicken	¾ c	70	4●	1●	11●	NA	NA	6○	6○	6○	2○	6○	*○	*○	4○
Cup-a-soup, green pea	¾ c	120	4●	4●	16●	NA	698○	*○	30●	6○	2○	2○	*○	2○	*○
Cup-a-soup, ring noodle	¾ c	50	2○	1●	9○	NA	1066○	*○	6○	2○	4○	4○	*○	*○	2○
Cup-a-soup, spring vegetable	¾ c	40	2○	1●	7○	NA	795○	4○	2○	*○	2○	4○	*○	*○	2○
Cup-a-soup, onion	¾ c	30	1○	1●	5○	NA	588○	*○	*○	*○	*○	*○	*○	*○	*○
Cup-a-soup, tomato	¾ c	80	1○	1●	17●	NA	630○	*○	*○	*○	*○	2○	4○	2○	2○
French onion, Campbell	1 c	70	2○	3●	9○	NA	990○	*○	2○	2○	2○	2○	2○	2○	*○
Minestrone, Campbell	1 c	80	3○	2●	11●	NA	960○	50●	2○	2○	2○	4○	2○	2○	2○
Onion, from mix	1 c	35	1○	1●	6○	NA	689○	58○	*○	*○	*○	*○	3○	1○	1○

Soups, Prep As Directed, cont'd.

Food	Serving	Calories	Protein g	Fat g	Carbo g	Fiber g	Sodium mg	Potassium mg	Vit A %rda	Vit B1 %rda (thiamin)	Vit B2 %rda (riboflavin)	Vit B3 %rda (niacin)	Vit C %rda	Calcium %rda	Iron %rda
Pea w/ham & bacon Campbell	1 c	170	8●	4●	24●	NA	850○	NA	6○	6○	2○	4○	*○	*○	10●
Split pea	1 c	145	9●	3●	21●	NA	967○	270●	9○	17●	9○	8○	2○	3○	8○
Tomato Campbell	1 c	90	1○	2●	17●	NA	760○	NA	6○	*○	*○	4○	2○	*○	2○
Tomato, low-sodium Campbell	1 cn	140	2○	4●	24●	NA	40●	NA	10○	*○	2○	6○	45●	4○	2○
Turkey noodle, low-sodium Campbell	1 cn	70	3○	3●	8○	NA	50●	NA	*○	*○	2○	6○	40●	4○	4○
Vegetable Campbell	1 c	80	2○	2●	12●	NA	770○	NA	50●	2○	*○	4○	*○	*○	2○
Vegetable beef, low-sodium Campbell	1 cn	90	6●	4●	9○	NA	60●	NA	50●	*○	*○	4○	*○	4○	4○
Vegetable, low-sodium Campbell	1 cn	90	3○	2●	15●	NA	50●	NA	45●	*○	*○	4○	*○	*○	2○
Vegetarian vegetable Campbell	1 c	70	1○	2●	12●	NA	790○	NA	50●	2○	*○	2○	2○	*○	2○

TV Dinners

Food	Serving	Calories	Protein g	Fat g	Carbo g	Fiber g	Sodium mg	Potassium mg	Vit A %rda	Vit B1 %rda (thiamin)	Vit B2 %rda (riboflavin)	Vit B3 %rda (niacin)	Vit C %rda	Calcium %rda	Iron %rda
Chicken, fried, white meat Hungry-Man	1	950	43	47	90	NA	1935	NA	*	35	25	70	15	10	25
Chicken, fried, white meat Swanson	1	570	29	29	48	NA	1395	NA	10	15	15	30	15	4	15
Fish 'n chips Hungry-Man	1	820	30	39	87	NA	1585	NA	10	40	30	25	10	6	25
Fish 'n chips Swanson	1	460	22	22	43	NA	925	NA	*	10	15	15	20	2	10
Lasagne w/meat Hungry-Man	1	690	24	26	90	NA	1485	NA	6	50	40	30	30	25	40
Salisbury steak Hungry-Man	1	780	34	43	63	NA	1800	NA	*	30	30	45	25	8	35
Salisbury steak Swanson	1	430	16	21	43	NA	1345	NA	*	10	10	15	15	4	10
Sliced beef Hungry-Man	1	500	38	15	55	NA	1345	NA	10	10	20	40	25	4	25
Spaghetti w/meatballs Swanscn	1	370	11	16	46	NA	1065	NA	15	10	10	15	40	10	5

TV Dinners, cont'd.

Food	Serving	Calories	Protein g	Fat g	Carbo g	Fiber g	Sodium mg	Potassium mg	Vit A % rda	Vit B1 % rda (thiamin)	Vit B2 % rda (riboflavin)	Vit B3 % rda (niacin)	Vit C % rda	Calcium % rda	Iron % rda
Turkey Hungry-Man	1	600 ●	37 ●	19 ○	70 ●	NA	2045	NA	* ○	35 ●	25 ●	50 ●	30 ●	6 ○	30 ●
Turkey Swanson	1	340 ●	19 ●	15 ○	40 ●	NA	1200 ○	NA	60 ●	15 ●	10 ●	30 ●	15 ○	4 ○	10 ●
Veal parmigiana Hungry-Man	1	700 ●	35 ●	34 ○	61 ●	NA	2190	NA	25 ●	30 ●	30 ●	40 ●	45 ●	20 ○	20 ●
Veal parmigiana Swanson	1	450 ●	22 ●	20 ○	46 ●	NA	970 ○	NA	* ○	15 ●	20 ●	35 ●	30 ●	8 ○	15 ●

Fast Food
Fast Food Breakfast Items

Food	Serving	Calories	Protein g	Fat g	Carbo g	Fiber g	Sodium mg	Potassium mg	Vit A %rda	Vit B1 %rda (thiamin)	Vit B2 %rda (riboflavin)	Vit B3 %rda (niacin)	Vit C %rda	Calcium %rda	Iron %rda
Biscuit w/jelly Hardee's	1 pr	324	5	13	48	NA	653	131	*	23	14	4	*	15	15
Biscuit w/sausage Burger Chef	1 pr	418	16	25	33	NA	1313	326	1	47	24	22	2	16	11
Biscuit, ham Hardee's	1 pr	349	12	17	37	NA	1415	235	3	40	29	9	*	18	18
Biscuit, sausage Hardee's	1 pr	413	10	26	34	NA	864	217	*	24	13	14	*	14	15
Biscuit, steak Hardee's	1 pr	419	14	23	41	NA	804	265	*	23	25	16	*	12	26
Breakfast Jack	1	300	18	13	28	NA	1035	NA	8	25	30	25	6	20	15
Egg & bacon Burger Chef	1 pr	567	21	31	50	NA	1108	574	11	27	29	18	NA	15	22
Egg & sausage Burger Chef	1 pr	668	26	40	50	NA	1411	688	11	47	35	25	7	16	23
Egg McMuffin	1	327	19	15	31	NA	885	NA	12	31	26	19	2	23	16
Eggs breakfast Jack-in-the-Box	1 pr	720	26	44	55	NA	1110	NA	15	45	35	25	20	25	30
Eggs, scrambled McDonald's	1 pr	180	13	13	3	NA	205	NA	13	5	28	*	2	6	14

Fast Food Breakfast Items, cont'd.

Food	Serving	Calories	Protein g	Fat g	Carbo g	Fiber g	Sodium mg	Potassium mg	Vit A %rda	Vit B1 %rda (thiamin)	Vit B2 %rda (riboflavin)	Vit B3 %rda (niacin)	Vit C %rda	Calcium %rda	Iron %rda
Hotcakes McDonald's	1 pr	500	8	10	94	NA	1070	NA	5	17	21	11	8	10	12
Pancakes breakfast Jack-in-the-Box	1 pr	630	16	27	79	NA	1670	NA	10	40	25	25	45	10	15
Sausage, McDonald's	1 pr	206	9	19	1	NA	615	NA	NA	18	6	10	NA	*	5
Sunrise w/bacon Burger Chef	1 pr	392	19	21	30	NA	978	209	11	27	29	15	NA	19	18
Sunrise w/sausage Burger Chef	1 pr	526	26	33	30	NA	1412	350	11	47	35	24	2	20	21

Fast Food Desserts

Food	Serving	Calories	Protein g	Fat g	Carbo g	Fiber g	Sodium mg	Potassium mg	Vit A %rda	Vit B1 %rda (thiamin)	Vit B2 %rda (riboflavin)	Vit B3 %rda (niacin)	Vit C %rda	Calcium %rda	Iron %rda
Cookies McDonaldland	1 pr	308	4	11	49	NA	358	NA	*	15	14	14	*	8	8
Cookies, chocolaty chip McDonald's	1 pr	342	4	16	45	NA	313	NA	*	8	13	9	*	3	9
Sundae, caramel McDonald's	1	328	7	10	53	0	195	6	6	4	18	5	20	20	*

Fast Food Desserts, cont'd.

Food	Serving	Calories	Protein g	Fat g	Carbo g	Fiber g	Sodium mg	Potassium mg	Vit A % rda	Vit B1 % rda (thiamin)	Vit B2 % rda (riboflavin)	Vit B3 % rda (niacin)	Vit C % rda	Calcium % rda	Iron % rda
Sundae, hot fudge McDonald's	1	310	7	11	46	0	175	NA	5	4	18	6	4	22	3
Sundae, strawberry McDonald's	1	289	6	9	46	0	96	NA	6	4	17	5	5	17	2
Turnover, apple Hardee's	1	282	3	14	37	NA	NA	17	*	2	2	2	*	*	5
Turnover, apple Jack-in-the-Box	1	410	4	24	45	NA	350	NA	*	15	6	10	*	*	8
Turnover, lemon Jack-in-the-Box	1	450	4	26	49	NA	405	NA	*	15	6	15	*	*	8

Fast Food Pizza

Food	Serving	Calories	Protein g	Fat g	Carbo g	Fiber g	Sodium mg	Potassium mg	Vit A % rda	Vit B1 % rda (thiamin)	Vit B2 % rda (riboflavin)	Vit B3 % rda (niacin)	Vit C % rda	Calcium % rda	Iron % rda
Anchovy, Shakey's	2 sl	301	16	11	38	NA	NA	NA	NA	NA	NA	NA	NA	NA	NA
Beef & onion Shakey's	2 sl	327	22	11	37	NA	NA	NA	NA	NA	NA	NA	NA	NA	NA
Bullfighters Shakey's	2 sl	332	17	14	39	NA	NA	NA	NA	NA	NA	NA	NA	NA	NA
Canadian bacon Shakey's	2 sl	336	19	14	40	NA	NA	NA	NA	NA	NA	NA	NA	NA	NA

Fast Food Pizza, cont'd.

Food	Serving	Calories	Protein g	Fat g	Carbo g	Fiber g	Sodium mg	Potassium mg	Vit A %rda	Vit B1 %rda (thiamin)	Vit B2 %rda (riboflavin)	Vit B3 %rda (niacin)	Vit C %rda	Calcium %rda	Iron %rda
Cheese, Shakey's	2 sl	309	16●	12○	38●	NA	NA	NA	NA	NA	NA	NA	NA	NA	NA
Cheese, thick-crust Pizza Hut	2 sl	390	24●	10○	53●	NA	800○	290○	16○	50●	70●	40●	*○	60●	25●
Cheese, thin-crust Pizza Hut	2 sl	340	19●	11○	42●	NA	900○	190○	12○	30●	30●	20●	*○	50●	20●
Hawaiian Delight Shakey's	2 sl	345	19●	14○	43●	NA	NA	NA	NA	NA	NA	NA	NA	NA	NA
Idiot's delight Shakey's	2 sl	288	14●	10○	40●	NA	NA	NA	NA	NA	NA	NA	NA	NA	NA
Italian salami Shakey's	2 sl	345	18●	16○	38●	NA	NA	NA	NA	NA	NA	NA	NA	NA	NA
Italian sausage Shakey's	2 sl	334	22●	12○	38●	NA	NA	NA	NA	NA	NA	NA	NA	NA	NA
Mexican Fiesta Shakey's	2 sl	334	17●	14○	39●	NA	NA	NA	NA	NA	NA	NA	NA	NA	NA
Mushroom, Shakey's	2 sl	286	14●	10○	38●	NA	NA	NA	NA	NA	NA	NA	NA	NA	NA
Pepperoni, thick-crust Pizza Hut	2 sl	450	25●	16○	52●	NA	900○	300◐	30◐	55●	40●	25●	*○	50●	25●

Fast Food Pizza, cont'd.

Food	Serving	Calories	Protein, g	Fat, g	Carbo, g	Fiber, g	Sodium, mg	Potassium, mg	Vit A %rda	Vit B1 %rda (thiamin)	Vit B2 %rda (riboflavin)	Vit B3 %rda (niacin)	Vit C %rda	Calcium %rda	Iron %rda
Pepperoni, thin-crust Pizza Hut	2 sl	370	19	15	42	NA	1000	225	14	30	25	20	*	40	18
Pork-mushroom, thick-crust Pizza Hut	2 sl	430	27	14	53	NA	1000	420	20	60	35	55	4	40	30
Pork-mushroom, thin-crust Pizza Hut	2 sl	380	21	14	44	NA	1200	340	15	35	30	30	*	12	25
Royal Canadian Shakey's	2 sl	345	20	14	42	NA	NA	NA	NA	NA	NA	NA	NA	NA	NA
Shakey's special	2 sl	382	23	16	38	NA	NA	NA	NA	NA	NA	NA	NA	NA	NA
Smoked oyster Shakey's	2 sl	294	16	10	39	NA	NA	NA	NA	NA	NA	NA	NA	NA	NA
Super supreme, thick-crust Pizza Hut	2 sl	590	34	26	55	NA	1400	465	80	55	60	40	6	35	35
Super supreme, thin-crust Pizza Hut	2 sl	520	30	26	46	NA	1500	415	70	40	40	40	6	30	30

Fast Food Pizza, cont'd.

Food	Serving	Calories	Protein g	Fat g	Carbo g	Fiber g	Sodium mg	Potassium mg	Vit A %rda	Vit B1 %rda (thiamin)	Vit B2 %rda (riboflavin)	Vit B3 %rda (niacin)	Vit C %rda	Calcium %rda	Iron %rda
Supreme, thick-crust Pizza Hut	2 sl	480 ●	29 ●	18 ○	52 ●	NA	1000 ○	405 ●	20 ●	60 ●	45 ●	50 ●	6 ○	55 ●	30 ●
Supreme, thin-crust Pizza Hut	2 sl	400 ●	21 ●	17 ○	44 ●	NA	1200 ○	335 ●	15 ●	45 ●	30 ●	30 ●	4 ○	40 ●	25 ●

Fast Food Platters

Food	Serving	Calories	Protein g	Fat g	Carbo g	Fiber g	Sodium mg	Potassium mg	Vit A %rda	Vit B1 %rda (thiamin)	Vit B2 %rda (riboflavin)	Vit B3 %rda (niacin)	Vit C %rda	Calcium %rda	Iron %rda
Chicken McNuggets	1 pr	314 ●	20 ●	19 ○	15 ○	NA	525 ○	* ○	8 ○	9 ○	43 ●	3 ○	* ○	6 ○
Chicken Planks LJ Silvers	4 pc	457 ●	27 ●	23 ○	35 ●	NA	NA	NA	NA	NA	NA	NA	NA	NA
Chili, Wendy's	1 pr	230 ●	19 ●	8 ○	21 ●	NA	1065 ○	20 ●	10 ●	10 ●	15 ●	4 ○	8 ○	20 ●
Clams, breaded LJ Silvers	1 pr	617 ●	18 ●	34 ○	61 ●	NA	NA	NA	NA	NA	NA	NA	NA	NA
Fish w/batter LJ Silvers	2 pc	366 ●	22 ●	22 ○	21 ●	NA	NA	NA	NA	NA	NA	NA	NA	NA
Fun meal Burger Chef	1 pr	514 ●	14 ●	19 ●	85 ●	NA	615 ○	2 ○	27 ●	12 ●	24 ●	16 ○	8 ○	17 ●

Fast Food Platters, cont'd.

Food	Serving	Calories	Protein g	Fat g	Carbo g	Fiber g	Sodium mg	Potassium mg	Vit A %rda	Vit B1 %rda (thiamin)	Vit B2 %rda (riboflavin)	Vit B3 %rda (niacin)	Vit C %rda	Calcium %rda	Iron %rda
Oysters, breaded LJ Silvers	6 pc	441●	13○	19●	53●	NA	NA	NA	NA	NA	NA	NA	NA	NA	NA
Peg Legs LJ Silvers	5 pc	350●	22●	28●	26●	NA	NA	NA	NA	NA	NA	NA	NA	NA	NA
Scallops, ocean LJ Silvers	6 pc	283●	11○	13●	30●	NA	NA	NA	NA	NA	NA	NA	NA	NA	NA
Shrimp w/batter LJ Silvers	6 pc	268●	8○	13●	30●	NA	NA	NA	NA	NA	NA	NA	NA	NA	NA
Treasure Chest LJ Silvers	1 pr	506●	30●	33●	32●	NA	NA	NA	NA	NA	NA	NA	NA	NA	NA

Fast Food Sandwiches

Food	Serving	Calories	Protein g	Fat g	Carbo g	Fiber g	Sodium mg	Potassium mg	Vit A %rda	Vit B1 %rda (thiamin)	Vit B2 %rda (riboflavin)	Vit B3 %rda (niacin)	Vit C %rda	Calcium %rda	Iron %rda
Beef and cheese Arby's	1	450●	27●	22●	36●	NA	1220○	NA	*○	25●	25●	30●	*○	20●	25●
Big Deluxe Hardee's	1	546●	29●	26●	48●	NA	1083●	594●	8○	33●	43●	53●	71●	10○	37●
Big Mac	1	563●	26●	33●	41●	NA	1010○	NA	11○	26●	22●	32●	4○	16○	22●
Big Shef	1	556●	22●	36●	37●	NA	840○	267●	6○	27●	24●	30●	3○	18○	20●

Fast Food Sandwiches, cont'd.

Food	Serving	Calories	Protein g	Fat g	Carbo g	Fiber g	Sodium mg	Potassium mg	Vit A %rda	Vit B1 %rda (thiamin)	Vit B2 %rda (riboflavin)	Vit B3 %rda (niacin)	Vit C %rda	Calcium %rda	Iron %rda
Cheeseburger Burger Chef	1	278	14	12	28	NA	641	162	5	20	18	18	2	15	13
Cheeseburger Hardee's	1	335	17	17	29	NA	789	197	15	34	19	27	*	5	15
Cheeseburger Jack-in-the-Box	1	310	16	15	28	NA	875	A	6	20	10	25	*	15	15
Cheeseburger McDonald's	1	307	15	14	30	NA	767	NA	7	17	14	19	3	13	13
Cheeseburger w/bacon supreme Jack-in-the-Box	1	790	33	54	43	NA	NA	NA	6	35	35	45	6	30	30
Cheeseburger, double Burger Chef	1	402	23	22	28	NA	835	244	8	20	24	26	2	22	16
Chicken supreme Jack-in-the-Box	1	700	28	45	47	NA	NA	NA	4	30	20	50	15	25	20
Club supreme Jack-in-the-Box	1	426	20	22	37	NA	NA	NA	*	39	19	26	55	21	12
Double cheese Wendy's	1	800	50	48	41	NA	1414	NA	8	30	40	50	2	15	50
Double, Wendy's	1	670	44	40	34	NA	980	NA	2	25	30	50	2	10	45

Fast Food Sandwiches, cont'd.

Food	Serving	Calories	Protein g	Fat g	Carbo g	Fiber g	Sodium mg	Potassium mg	Vit A %rda	Vit B1 %rda (thiamin)	Vit B2 %rda (riboflavin)	Vit B3 %rda (niacin)	Vit C %rda	Calcium %rda	Iron %rda
Filet-o-fish McDonald's	1	432	14	25	37	NA	781	NA	4	18	12	13	NA	9	10
Fish, big Hardee's	1	514	20	26	49	NA	314	290	23	NA	89	36	8	9	29
Ham & cheese Hardee's	1	376	23	15	37	NA	1067	317	4	24	44	13	*	21	21
Ham & cheese supreme Jack-in-the-Box	1	500	31	22	42	NA	NA	NA	*	70	30	35	*	35	20
Hamburger Burger Chef	1	235	11	9	27	NA	480	144	2	20	12	18	2	8	12
Hamburger Hardee's	1	305	16	13	29	NA	682	231	*	37	34	32	*	2	20
Hamburger Jack-in-the-Box	1	260	13	11	29	NA	565	NA	*	20	10	25	2	8	15
Hamburger McDonald's	1	255	12	10	30	NA	520	NA	*	16	11	20	3	5	13
Hot dog, Hardee's	1	346	11	22	26	NA	744	120	*	19	13	21	*	4	14
Jumbo Jack	1	550	28	29	45	NA	1135	NA	4	30	20	60	6	15	25

Fast Food Sandwiches, cont'd.

Food	Serving	Calories	Protein g	Fat g	Carbo g	Fiber g	Sodium mg	Potassium mg	Vit A %rda	Vit B1 %rda (thiamin)	Vit B2 %rda (riboflavin)	Vit B3 %rda (niacin)	Vit C %rda	Calcium %rda	Iron %rda
Jumbo Jack w/cheese	1	630●	32●	35○	45●	NA	1665○	NA	15○	35●	20●	60●	8○	25●	25●
Junior, Arby's	1	220●	12●	9○	21●	NA	530○	434●	*○	10●	10●	15●	*○	4○	10●
Moby Jack	1	450●	17●	26○	38●	NA	835○	NA	4○	20●	10●	20●	*○	15●	8○
Mushroom burger Burger Chef	1	520●	28●	29○	34●	NA	744●	434●	7○	27●	35●	40●	5○	26●	21●
Quarter Pounder McDonald's	1	424●	24●	22○	33●	NA	735○	NA	3○	21●	17●	32●	NA	6○	23●
Quarter Pounder w/cheese McDonald's	1	524●	30●	31○	32●	NA	1236●	NA	13○	21●	22●	37●	5○	22●	24●
Roast beef Hardee's	1	377●	21●	17○	36●	NA	1030●	205●	11○	62●	11●	19●	5○	6○	35●
Roast beef, Arby's	1	350●	22●	15○	32●	NA	880●	NA	*○	20●	20●	25●	*○	8○	20●
Roast beef, big Hardee's	1	418●	28●	19○	34●	NA	1770○	470●	13○	69●	13●	26●	13○	7○	45●
Single cheese Wendy's	1	580●	33●	34○	34●	NA	1085●	NA	4○	25●	25●	30●	*○	20●	25●

Fast Food Sandwiches, cont'd.

Food	Serving	Calories	Protein g	Fat g	Carbo g	Fiber g	Sodium mg	Potassium mg	Vit A %rda	Vit B1 %rda (thiamin)	Vit B2 %rda (riboflavin)	Vit B3 %rda (niacin)	Vit C %rda	Calcium %rda	Iron %rda
Single, Wendy's	1	470	26	26	34	NA	774	*	15	20	25	*	8	25	
Super Shef	1	604	27	39	35	NA	1088	424	16	27	29	34	15	24	21
Super, Arby's	1	620	30	28	61	NA	1420	*	35	25	35	*	10	30	
Taco, regular Jack-in-the-Box	1	190	8	11	15	NA	460	6	4	4	8	*	10	10	6
Taco, super Jack-in-the-Box	1	280	12	17	20	NA	970	10	6	6	15	2	20	20	10
Triple cheese Wendy's	1	1040	72	68	35	NA	1848	8	50	45	70	4	35	60	
Triple, Wendy's	1	850	65	51	33	NA	1217	4	30	40	70	2	10	50	
Whopper	1	630	26	36	50	NA	990	520	*	4	15	20	4	10	15
Whopper Junior	1	370	15	20	31	NA	560	280	*	15	10	15	*	10	
Whopper w/cheese	1	740	32	45	52	NA	1435	590	*	8	20	15	15	15	
Whopper, double	1	850	44	52	52	NA	1080	760	*	6	25	30	2	2	25

Fast Food Sandwiches, cont'd.

Food	Serving	Calories	Protein g	Fat g	Carbo g	Fiber g	Sodium mg	Potassium mg	Vit A % rda	Vit B1 % rda (thiamin)	Vit B2 % rda (riboflavin)	Vit B3 % rda (niacin)	Vit C % rda	Calcium % rda	Iron % rda
Whopper, double w/cheese	1	950	50 ●	60 ○	54 ●	NA	1535 ○	730 ●	* ○	6 ○	25 ●	30 ●	* ○	15 ●	20 ●
Whopper Junior w/cheese	1	420	18 ●	25 ○	32 ●	NA	785 ○	270 ●	* ○	15 ●	10 ●	15 ●	* ○	8 ○	10 ○

Fast Food Shakes

Food	Serving	Calories	Protein g	Fat g	Carbo g	Fiber g	Sodium mg	Potassium mg	Vit A % rda	Vit B1 % rda (thiamin)	Vit B2 % rda (riboflavin)	Vit B3 % rda (niacin)	Vit C % rda	Calcium % rda	Iron % rda
Chocolate Burger Chef	1	403	10 ●	9 ○	72 ○	0	378 ○	762 ●	6 ○	13 ●	47 ●	2 ○	* ○	45 ●	3 ○
Chocolate McDonald's	1	383	10 ●	9 ○	66 ○	0	300 ●	NA	7 ○	8 ○	26 ●	3 ○	* ○	32 ●	5 ○
Frosty, Wendy's	1	390	9 ●	16 ●	54 ○	0	247 ●	NA	6 ○	10 ●	35 ●	5 ○	* ○	25 ●	
Milkshake, Hardee's	1	391	11 ●	10 ○	63 ○	0	NA	652 ●	* ○	13 ●	46 ●	3 ○	* ○	45 ●	4 ○
Shake, chocolate Burger King	1	340	8 ●	10 ●	57 ○	0	280 ●	340 ●	* ○	8 ○	15 ●	* ○	* ○	25 ●	
Shake, vanilla Burger King	1	340	8 ●	11 ●	52 ○	0	320 ●	210 ●	* ○	10 ●	20 ●	* ○	* ○	30 ●	* ○
Strawberry McDonald's	1	362	9 ●	9 ○	62 ○	0	207 ●	NA	8 ○	8 ○	26 ●	7 ○	* ○	32 ●	* ○

Fast Food Shakes, cont'd.

Food	Serving	Calories	Protein g	Fat g	Carbo g	Fiber g	Sodium mg	Potassium mg	Vit A %rda	Vit B1 %rda (thiamin)	Vit B2 %rda (riboflavin)	Vit B3 %rda (niacin)	Vit C %rda	Calcium %rda	Iron %rda
Vanilla Burger Chef	1	380	13	10	60	0	325	622	8	7	41	3	*	50	2
Vanilla, McDonald's	1	352	9	8	60	0	201	NA	7	8	41	*	5	33	*

Fast Food Vegetables

Food	Serving	Calories	Protein g	Fat g	Carbo g	Fiber g	Sodium mg	Potassium mg	Vit A %rda	Vit B1 %rda (thiamin)	Vit B2 %rda (riboflavin)	Vit B3 %rda (niacin)	Vit C %rda	Calcium %rda	Iron %rda
French Fryes LJ Silvers	1 pr	288	4	16	33	NA	NA	NA	NA	NA	NA	NA	NA	NA	NA
French fries Burger Chef	1 pr	204	3	10	26	NA	469	NA	7	*	6	12	1	4	4
French fries Jack-in-the-Box	1 pr	270	3	15	31	NA	130	*	8	*	10	6	2	2	4
French fries Wendy's	1 pr	330	5	16	41	NA	112	*	8	4	15	10	*	*	6
French fries, regular Burger King	1 pr	210	3	11	25	NA	230	*	4	4	4	4	*	*	2
French fries, small Hardee's	1 pr	239	3	13	28	NA	121	*	5	5	5	17	*	*	5
Fries, regular McDonald's	1 pr	220	3	12	26	NA	109	NA	8	8	11	21	*	3	3

Fast Food Vegetables, cont'd.

Food	Serving	Calories	Protein g	Fat g	Carbo g	Fiber g	Sodium mg	Potassium mg	Vit A %rda	Vit B1 %rda (thiamin)	Vit B2 %rda (riboflavin)	Vit B3 %rda (niacin)	Vit C %rda	Calcium %rda	Iron %rda
Hash browns McDonald's	1 pr	125	2	7	14	NA	325	NA	*	4	NA	4	7	*	5
Hasn rounds Burger Chef	1 pr	235	3	14	26	NA	349	434	7	7	*	7	6	1	5
Onion rings Jack-in-the-Box	1 pr	350	5	23	32	NA	320	NA	15	15	6	15	2	2	8
Onion rings, reg Burger King	1 pr	270	3	16	29	NA	450	140	4	4	*	*	*	8	2

About the Author

Patricia Hausman is author of two widely acclaimed books: *Foods That Fight Cancer* (Rawson Associates, 1984) and *Jack Sprat's Legacy: The Science and Politics of Fat and Cholesterol* (Richard Marek, 1981). She holds a Master's degree in nutrition from the University of Maryland and a Bachelor's degree in biology from Kirkland College.

She formerly served as staff nutritionist at the Center for Science in the Public Interest and was editor of its monthly magazine, *Nutrition Action*, for several years.

A frequent guest on radio and TV shows, she lives in Silver Spring, Maryland.